Monsignor William B. O'Brien
and Ellis Henican

YOU
CAN'T
DO IT
ALONE

THE DAYTOP WAY

TO MAKE YOUR

CHILD DRUG FREE

SIMON & SCHUSTER
New York   London
Toronto   Sydney
Tokyo   Singapore

SIMON & SCHUSTER
Simon & Schuster Building
Rockefeller Center
1230 Avenue of the Americas
New York, New York 10020

SIMON & SCHUSTER and colophon are registered trademarks of
Simon & Schuster Inc.
Designed by Pei Loi Koay
Manufactured in the United States of America

10 9 8 7 6 5 4 3 2 1

Library of Congress Cataloging-in-Publication Data

O'Brien, William B.
You can't do it alone: the Daytop way to make your child drug
free / Monsignor William B. O'Brien and Ellis Henican.
p.   cm.
Includes index.
1. Narcotic addicts—Rehabilitation.   2. Daytop Village, inc.
3. Therapeutic community.   I. Henican, Ellis.   II. Title.
HV5801.025   1993
362.29'18—dc20   93-22051
                                                           CIP

ISBN 0-671-72837-7

To the members of the Daytop family

who have inspired and enriched us

with their love, their courage, and

their incredible perseverance.

ACKNOWLEDGMENTS

This book could not have been written without the generosity and patience of the residents, graduates, and staff of Daytop Village. There is no use pretending otherwise. These brave people opened their hearts to us, sharing the often-painful details of their lives before, during, and after treatment. Their families and friends were similarly open and frank. It is our sincerest hope that this rugged honesty will be an inspiration to others.

Several Daytop staff members were extraordinarily helpful in the creation of this book, and they deserve special mention. Brian Madden, Daytop's executive vice-president, displayed infinite patience and a passion for detail. Vice-President Patricia Zingale always knew where to find what. Of course, she had first-rate backup from executive assistants Mary DeStio, Corinne Beveridge, and Linda Lehman. Cleo Odzer, special assistant to the president, was another immensely gifted researcher.

Charles Devlin—Daytop resident, graduate, and now vice-president—shared invaluable recollections from the early days, as did Robert Boriello and Vice-President David Deitch. It was Deitch who added the inspiration-dimension to Daytop's philosophy of treatment and prevention, and he still speaks in inspiring terms.

Vice-President Yasser Hijasi truly understands the mechanics of the Daytop organization. Research Director Vincent Biasi, the man who keeps the numbers, is able to interpret them in remarkably plain English. Roxy and Berge Kalijian, the angels of the Daytop

Family Association, can explain with wonderful clarity how families fit into all of this.

A long overdue thank-you must go to Alexander Bassin of Florida State University and to Joseph Shelly, retired chief of probation, second department, New York State. Without their vision, there would be no Daytop as we know it today. All these years later, both men were generous with their memories.

Finally, we are indebted to Dominick Anfuso and Casandra Jones at Simon & Schuster and to our agents, Philippa Brophy and William Spruill, at Sterling Lord Literistic. In the most practical ways, they made this book happen.

—W. B. O'B. and E. H.

CONTENTS

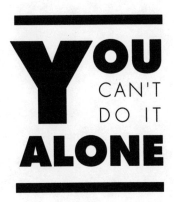

BROKEN HEARTS AND BROKEN DREAMS 1

The child is always innocent. / Each child needs among other things: care, protection, security, warmth, skin contact, touching, caressing, and tenderness. / These needs are seldom sufficiently fulfilled, and in fact they are often exploited by adults for their own ends (trauma of child abuse). / Child abuse has lifelong effects. Society takes the side of the adult and blames the child for what has been done to him or her. / The victimization of the child has historically been denied and is still being denied, even today. / This denial has made it possible for society to ignore the devastating effects of the victimization of the child for such a long time. / The child, when betrayed by society, has no choice but to repress the trauma and to idealize the abuser.

—Alice Miller, *Society's Betrayal of the Child*

My name is Timothy. I am twenty years old. We have three kids in my family—my older brother, my little sister and me. When we were little—I was, like, six at the time—my mother left us. She and my father weren't getting along. She was drinking too much, and she was seeing this shrink, a psychiatrist. And I guess she decided she fell in love with the shrink. So she decided to move out to California with him. That left the three of us with just my father.

Now, he didn't know much about raising kids. He was a cop in the city. I guess he was pretty upset about my mother running off like that. Anyway, he hired this lady to take care of us, and she was with us for, maybe, three years.

When I was nine, my mother called us on the telephone one day, and she said she missed her kids, and we should come out to California and visit her for Christmas.

I was still mad at her for leaving us and all. But I was also happy because she wanted us to come there. I can remember my sister and

*my brother and me being on the plane to San Francisco, talking
and being really excited about the trip.*

*My mother wasn't with the psychiatrist anymore. She was living by
herself. When we got out there, all four of us were crying about how
good it was to see each other. And we had a really nice Christmas.
We got a lot of presents. But mostly, it was just being with my mother
again. She told us how much she missed us, how much she hated
being separated by all those miles.*

*And then, two days after Christmas, she said she was going to come
back to New York with us, so we could all be near each other again.
"A mother shouldn't be away from her children. It isn't right." That's
what she said.*

*Then, what happened was we all went out to the airport to get
the plane to New York. We checked in at the counter, gave the airline
all the luggage, with the presents and everything.*

*I remember, we were walking out to the gate area, the four of us,
holding hands, family again. But then right at the last minute, my
mother changed her mind. Just as we were supposed to get on the
plane, she started crying. And she gave my brother all the tickets. She
said she couldn't do it. And she turned around and ran away.*

*The people from United Airlines didn't really know what to do.
They asked us if we had someone who was meeting us in New York,
and they let us get on the plane. They were real nice to us because
I think they knew what had happened and they felt really bad. The
three of us were crying all the way back.*

*Anyway, we went back and kept living with my father. You should
have heard how mad he was—he was screaming and throwing
stuff—when he heard about what my mother did.*

*After that, he got really strict with us, rigid about everything. It was
like he never got over being mad at my mother. Before he would go
off to work in the city, he would write up a list of all these chores
we were supposed to do and put them up on the refrigerator. He
didn't really talk to us too much. All he wanted to know was whether
we had done those chores. If anything was the least bit out of order,
he would start screaming and he would go on like that for the rest
of the night. Sometimes, he would get violent, too.*

*We had a few different housekeepers who looked after us. Some-
times, it was one of his girlfriends. Sometimes the housekeepers became his girlfriends.*

*But it was about four years later when we heard from my mother
again. She called us one day and said she finally did move back
East. She was living in Connecticut with her new boyfriend. She
wanted us to come up and see her.*

So we started going up there.

*It was kind of strange at first. I don't think my father really liked
the idea of us going up to Connecticut. But she was our mother,
you know. And it took some of the pressure off of him. My older
brother, he was still pretty mad at my mother, and the two of them
didn't really get along too well. He had started getting high, and he
was kind of moving away from the family. But for my sister and
me, it was the best of all possible worlds. We would see my mother
on weekends, be with my father during the week.*

*It was like this for almost two years. Then, one day we just got
this call.*

*My father was at work. My older brother answered the phone, and
he got this horrible look on his face, like when you know something
really bad has happened.*

*It was the state police in Connecticut. My mother got into a car
accident. The car was all bashed up, and my mother was killed.*

*The day after her funeral was the day I smoked reefer for the first
time. I made my brother give me some. You could probably say that
was the day I lost it. And for me, it was a long slide down.*

*My name is Christopher. I'm twenty-one years old. I grew up in a
pretty nice neighborhood in a suburb outside Dallas. I was the kind
of person that nobody would have guessed had a problem with drugs.
Nobody would have guessed I had any problems at all. I had a lot
of friends. I did okay in school. I had a family that was behind me
100 percent in anything I wanted to do. But the way things turned
out—anything my family was behind, I didn't want to have anything
to do with.*

I started getting high about ten years ago, when I was eleven. I was the youngest in my family, and all my brothers and sisters were getting high. It seemed like that's when they started to get their freedom from my parents.

They started getting high, smoking pot, going out all night, and they could do whatever it is they wanted. That's how I picked it up. I started smoking pot, doing what I wanted, drinking. It was like that through the seventh and eighth grades.

That's when my parents first saw a difference in me. They thought it was a phase, like with my brothers and sisters. Since I was the youngest I was just starting my phase before they started theirs. By the time I was seventeen, I had moved out of my house. By the time I was eighteen, I had a heart attack, off of getting some bad coke. Or, I don't know what it was, but I had a heart attack. I woke up one morning, and I was doing coke. That was normal for me. If I had any coke left, I wanted to do it right when I woke up in the morning. So I was just standing there with some friends, some people in my apartment, and I did the coke, and I just had a heart attack. That's when it all came out that I had a problem bigger than anybody thought.

When I had the heart attack, I got put in the hospital. I gave my sister some of the drugs that I had, although I still had more hidden. I made it look like, "Okay, this is what I have," when I realized I really had a lot more. I had to lay up in the hospital for a while, and I remember thinking, like, this is just too boring, being in here. So I got one of my friends to bring over the rest of my drugs. The doctor would come to see me, and I was still doing drugs. Two days after I had a heart attack. My heart got worse. The doctor knew. He told my parents. Everybody was screaming at each other. Everything got kind of crazy for a while. But when I got out of the hospital, I went back to my apartment, and things just kept on like they were.

When I was a kid I got hit by a car. I wasn't hurt too bad, but I had a lawsuit. And when I turned eighteen, I got money from the lawsuit. I got $50,000, and I ended up just blowing it, partying, because I wanted to lead the kind of life like in the movies—you know, just party all the time, just have your friends over to your apartment, just buy, buy, buy and never take responsibilities or *anything. It wasn't fun. Watching it on TV was a lot more fun than living it myself. Going on four-day runs, no sleep, then sleeping for twenty-four, thirty hours at a time, after you just passed out somewhere. Hurting everybody, pushing everybody in my family away from me.*

I didn't go home for Christmas, New Year's, my birthday, Easter, anything like that. I spent them all in my apartment by myself, feeling it all, feeling so lonely, feeling like I blew everything, like I'd burnt every bridge. I didn't have my friends. I didn't trust them. I didn't have my family because I burnt them. They tried to help me, and I was like, no, I didn't want their help. And with everybody else, it was a hush-hush kind of thing. Nobody expected this from Chris. It's like, "No, Chris couldn't lead that kind of life. I thought he was doing so good."

My name is LaShanda. I'm eighteen years old. I was born in Washington, D.C. I moved to New York with my mother and my sister when I was three years old because my mother and father separated. He was beating up on my mother and things. So we moved here. My mother was on welfare, so we had to do a lot of things to struggle so we could get by.

My mother was an alcoholic. When I was younger, my mother's friends used to come over, and they used to be drunk and everything. It wasn't too much fun for me. Like the males, some of them would abuse me and stuff. I would never tell my mother. When she was drunk, she would always be wanting to fight. And I didn't want my mother to be fighting no men, so I would never tell my mother these men was touching on me and things like that.

I let it go for all these years. I was, maybe, eight, nine, ten. They used to tell me, "You sit on my lap. I'll buy you a pair of roller skates." I wanted things like other kids, so I would do it, you know? I thought I would get something, even though I never did.

Before I came into Daytop, I was getting high on crack. I got high every single day of the week. I stole things. I robbed from people. One time I stole a ring, an engagement ring from my friend's mother, and I sold that. I was living with a sixty-year-old man, who used to buy my drugs. He supported my crack habit for a year. And I lived with him. I went from his house to my boyfriend's house, from his house to my boyfriend's house. Whenever I wanted to get high, I would go to him and I would let him have sex with me, you know, so I could get drugs.

I was just wasting away. I knew I could be doing better. I didn't really like myself anymore. I blamed myself for a lot of things. My family's problems, I thought, I was the cause of. I thought my mother was drinking because of me. I figured if I wasn't there, a lot of things wouldn't go on.

When I was sixteen, my mother disowned me. At the time, she had stopped drinking. She was doing good. She was trying to do things for herself, and she didn't want to be bothered by me. I was getting high. I had dropped out of school in the ninth grade. For me, it was hard. You could say I was living on the streets. I was going from one place to the other. I had no steady place where I could call home anymore. I was lonely because all my friends stopped being bothered with me. I hit rock bottom. I didn't dress nice anymore. I didn't take showers and baths every day. I disrespected myself. I had a bad reputation in my neighborhood. Everybody knew my name, you know, when I would pass.

If these are the voices of our nation's young people, what kind of country are we living in? A recent survey of the attitudes and experiences of Americans offers some eye-opening clues.

Ninety-one percent of Americans admit to lying regularly. Just 13 percent believe in the Ten Commandments. One of every fourteen Americans would agree to murder for money. One of every seven was sexually abused as a child.

Sixty-eight percent of Americans say we have no more living heroes. Sixty percent have been the victim of a major crime. In fact, we have more crime than any country on Earth—a homicide rate five to twenty times that of any other industrialized nation. Forty-one percent of Americans admit to using drugs for fun. Drunk drivers are the number-one killers of Americans under forty, yet

58 percent of Americans admit to driving drunk. One in seven Americans carries a weapon. Forty-seven percent know someone who committed suicide. One of every three Americans would volunteer to pull the switch on an electric chair.

Clearly, something is very wrong out there. But we don't need statistics to tell us that. We experience the consequences every day.

We are living at a time of great moral and social crisis. The basic values that used to guide us—honesty; personal responsibility; a respect for hard work; a belief in God, family, and community— don't hold much sway anymore. And the problem isn't just that we are falling short of these traditional ideals. The problem goes deeper, I'm afraid. Many of us don't even *have* ideals anymore.

We try to convince ourselves that we can be happy in a kind of plush isolation. We look for comfort in material things—our high-status cars, our designer clothing, our electronic gear. To be sure, our society has made great advances in science, in medicine, in consumerism, in the myriad of ways we can now spend our leisure time.

But still, our families are falling apart.

The 50 percent divorce rate is only part of it. There's also the shockingly high incidence of wife-beating and child abuse and the silent sexual crimes that occur in who-knows-how-many American homes. But even in families that have managed to avoid these dramatic eruptions, a more pervasive kind of failure has taken hold: Many of us have all but given up trying to instill real values in our children. Instead, we send them off into a difficult world—at an earlier and earlier age—with few of the basic skills they need to survive. And then we are flabbergasted when we look at them and notice they are not living useful, happy lives.

Drug abuse. Crime. Depression. A permanent state of dependence. An adolescence that runs clear into middle age. Too many of our young people are truly dying before our eyes, or being gravely maimed. If you don't believe this, visit a prison. Or talk to the kids who are hanging out at the local shopping mall. Our neighborhoods have become battlegrounds and graveyards. Our American dream of a better life for our children is fading into a distant hope. We have invented nothing to replace those old, discarded values. We are genuinely in danger of being swallowed up.

And the biggest threat by far, the one that swallows more young lives than any other, is drug abuse.

How can we then be surprised when young people turn for solace to the numbing pleasure of recreational drugs? Crack, heroin, cocaine, pills: the particular chemicals aren't so important. What matters is the role these substances play in destroying the lives of our young. And some trendy, stop-gap measure like passing out free, antiseptic needles, I'm afraid, isn't going to hold back the tide.

Drugs are the ultimate scream of anguish by the young.

They are a very special brand of suicide that allows the victim-perpetrator to die slowly, so that the message of anguish and hopelessness can be drawn out over a good, long time.

But are we listening? There's precious little evidence that we are. The walls of our denial and inaction are far too high for that, and they are getting higher.

These young people skirt around our homes and the back alleys of our towns, dying one painful day at a time. And what do we do? We settle into our softest easy chair to watch the current law-and-order television show or the latest orchestrated drug bust and nod approvingly as gallant federal agents break down the door of some ramshackle bungalow and pin the unwitting inhabitants to the floor. One thing can spur us to action, though. The minute we hear the earliest rumor that a drug-recovery center may be opening in our community, we are out of the house in a flash and onto the front lines of screaming opposition.

The war on drugs, we call it. Hooray for us!

We have succeeded in glamorizing the good-guy-over-the-bad-guy syndrome and produced millions for television advertisers. But how much of a good guy am I when I do nothing to help the youngsters from my own home or from across the street who at this very moment are being propelled into drug-infested pizza parlors and video arcades where they hope to escape the horror and emptiness of everyday life?

No wonder young people turn to mind-numbing chemicals to survive.

We have taught our children to demand what we ourselves have come to expect: Instant gratification. Easy answers. Comfortable distance. The God-given right to avoid pain at any cost.

Look at the messages the advertising media send out: Escape through the fantasy of cinema. Escape through the sedatives of liquor and beer. Destroy your health with cigarettes. It's glamorous. Avoid all discomfort through the palliative of over-the-counter drugs.

Our kids are bombarded with the same greedy, consumer-driven content—at higher decibels—on the radio, on MTV, at concerts, and at clubs. This cacophony of voices, dripping in charm, tells them to *take more, have fun, get down, chill out and do it all with impunity.*

When the going gets tough, we and they expect the solutions to come from the outside: Wait for someone—anyone—to step forward with an easy answer, the kind we've all become accustomed to. "Why can't we buy some service like a doctor, a teacher or a therapist?" "Why can't I get the neighborhood shrink to put Johnny back together, the same way the orthopedic surgeon mended the latest football injury?" "Why can't the teachers do something about those drug-using schoolkids who are infecting my blameless Genevieve? Didn't we just increase their salaries by a third?" Why can't? Why can't? Why can't someone else do the work?

Even those parents who try to maintain a strong bulwark of values quickly discover what powerful forces are pulling the other way. A recent United Nations study found that parents exercise the primary influence over their children only up to age seven. After that, the peers take over. So here we have all these children bursting out of their shells into a world filled with double messages, fortified by double-standard parental role-modeling and sealed by the American rationale of success-at-any-cost.

Where are the real answers to come from?

Unfortunately, the psychiatrists and other licensed "experts" in the mental-health field have relatively little to offer drug-using kids in a valueless world. They don't have a clue because their "great father," Sigmund Freud, didn't have a clue. Freud knew psychosis and neurosis, and his professional descendants do know something about confronting those twin disorders. But drug and alcohol addiction generally don't fall into either of those categories. Addiction belongs in the "character-disorder" zone that Freud (who himself used cocaine to survive) never addressed.

To make matters worse, psychiatry shifted its emphasis in the second half of the twentieth century from family-produced rationales to biochemistry. This may be quite useful for treating schizophrenia or chemical depression. But when it comes to young drug abusers, this psychiatry-as-a-branch-of-pharmacology is way off the mark. These kids already come from a pharmacological wasteland. Drugs are not the answer for drug problems.

At the same time, the social institutions that should be stepping in to help have mostly looked the other way. Where are our leaders from government, from the churches and temples, from the schools and colleges, from entertainment and sports? Most of them are silent—the ones who aren't busy leading our young people *toward* drugs. And a handful of celebrity just-say-no commercials will never be enough to reverse this deadly fact.

For thirty years now, Daytop Village has been working to fill this void. Ours is the business, quite simply, of rebuilding young lives. Today, Daytop is the largest and oldest drug-treatment program of its kind in the United States. Since opening our doors in 1963, we have helped rescue seventy-five thousand drug abusers, and we've helped heal nearly as many fractured families along the way.

I say "helped" in both cases because, in the final analysis, turning a life around is something only that individual can do. But almost no one ever does it alone. What Daytop has provided for these seventy-five thousand drug abusers is the technique, the structure and the support for making real changes happen—and for making sure the changes last.

This involves much more than just separating addicts from their drugs. If genuine change is to be achieved, the whole person—the whole family—must be profoundly healed.

Daytop accomplishes this by teaching some old-fashioned values that, frequently, are just not taught today.

What Daytop does, in a very real sense, is to re-create the family and send the youngster through a second time. Only now, it's a healthy, nourishing family. And the young addict has a chance to learn the lessons that were missed that first time around.

The core of Daytop treatment is a network of eight "houses," located in rural settings, away from the pressures and influences of city life. These houses, run by Daytop-trained ex-addicts, become the young person's family for as long as it takes to strip down and rebuild. It could be ten months, twelve months, fourteen months or longer. At Daytop, no one progresses simply by putting in the time. Hard work and achievement are demanded of everyone. And there's no guarantee that you'll succeed. Some people don't, and they are shown the door.

These Daytop houses are highly structured places. Much time is spent in self-analysis and group therapy. All the residents are expected to help with the running of the house, and everyone has a job. New residents start with the most menial tasks—scrubbing pots, maybe, or shoveling snow. Only by demonstrating responsibility and self-discipline does the Daytop resident progress to more interesting and higher-status jobs.

For those who are less seriously addicted to drugs and self-destructive behavior, Daytop also creates this family environment on an out-patient, six-day-a-week basis in eight Outreach Centers.

Rules are taken seriously in the Daytop family, but there's a lot of love, as well. It's just a different kind of love from the one that many of these kids grew up with. It's not the love that says, "Do anything you want, it's all right with me." It's certainly not the love that says, "Here, let me show my love by giving you a pair of expensive sneakers or another video game or the keys to a new Jaguar." It is not, in other words, a consuming, destructive kind of love that gives young drug users permission to go out and destroy their lives.

The family we have created inside Daytop is built on a tough love, an honest love, a love that demands.

It's a love that says, "I love you so much I will let you earn your status and privileges." It is a love that says, "I will expect you to look out for one another and build faith in yourself."

These things might sound basic. They might even sound a little harsh. But the life skills that are allowed to flourish in such an environment can mean the difference between life and death for a recovering drug addict. Unless the ingrained cycle of irresponsibility is broken, these young people are depressingly likely to return to the safety and the numbness of drugs.

The basic concept behind Daytop treatment is called the therapeutic community. It is an extremely powerful tool that, when used correctly, can produce dramatic and long-lasting changes. This is not easy. And it requires real commitment. But it is truly a process to behold. One day, I am convinced, the usefulness of this powerful concept will be recognized far beyond the world of drug abuse.

Daytop does not succeed with everybody.

Some people who come to us are not ready to change, or refuse to engage in the self-analysis we demand of them, or are just not willing to work hard enough. But remarkably often, the Daytop approach produces results. We take in some of the most difficult, hard-core drug addicts anywhere, often after they have failed in other treatment programs. Five years after graduating from Daytop,

88 percent of our kids are drug free, crime free, and either working or in school.

These aren't just our numbers. Researchers from Johns Hopkins University recently performed an exhaustive investigation into the therapeutic community's methods and results. Their conclusions almost exactly paralleled ours.

It's a record we've maintained now for a solid three decades. For us, it is a cause of genuine pride.

- The 75,000 young people whose lives we have turned around.
- The 2,400 who are currently being treated at Daytop in New York, California, Texas, New Jersey, Florida and Pennsylvania.
- Our Family Therapy Program for the parents and siblings of addicts, which "heals broken families."
- Our leadership training in the thirty-two countries where Daytop-style recovery programs now exist, a great expansion of our "healing forces."
- The 3 million young addicts and family members who have joined this worldwide Daytop revolution.
- The 4 million people in America alone who have been a part of Daytop's drug-prevention activities—young people, parents, teachers, church leaders and others, attending Daytop speaking engagements, seminars, groups and workshops over twenty-eight years.
- The teaching we have provided through our Promethean Institute in Pennsylvania and our various publications, all hammering home the message that the family-in-crisis is the central issue behind drug abuse and that our world must be changed into a responsible, caring one.
- The role we've played in creating two important organizations, Therapeutic Communities of America, Inc., and the World Federation of Therapeutic Communities, Inc., both of which Daytop helped to found.

But we are getting a little ahead of our story here. For now, it is important just to know the roughest outlines of this thing called Daytop. In the pages that follow, I will try to explain why the Daytop approach has been proven so successful in a realm where many others have tried and failed. Thankfully, there are some lessons here that parents and teachers—and yes, young people themselves—can learn to incorporate into their lives.

First, however, we need to get grounded with a little history. It is a history of spectacular failure, as society came face to face with drug abuse. A major turning point in that history occurred on a beachfront in California, where a crazed but brilliant man stumbled onto a truly sensible idea.

But the story opens three thousand miles from there, on the East Coast of the United States, with a gruesome murder near a public swimming pool in New York City—and with the echoes that this crime created for one particular young Catholic priest.

MICHAEL FARMER IS DEAD 2

Care is a state in which something does matter, care is the opposite of apathy. Care is important because it is what is missing in our day. What young people have been fighting, in revolts on college campuses and in the sweep of protests about the world, is the seeping, creeping conviction that nothing matters; the prevailing feeling that we can't do any-thing. The threat is apathy, uninvolvement, the grasping for external stimulants as found in drugs. Care is a necessary antidote for this.

—Rollo May, *Love and Will*

Michael Farmer was killed in the summer of 1957 in a neighborhood called Washington Heights. Even now, after all these years, the story sends chills down my back. Farmer was fifteen years old that summer, the oldest son of a city fireman. As police told the story, he was sliced open with a machete, stabbed with a hunting knife and then beaten with a wooden club, a lead-weighted dog chain, a studded belt, and several pairs of fists. His body was found in a clump of bushes near the public swimming pool at Highbridge Park.

Nineteen fifty-seven was a tense time all over New York. Money was tight. Racial attitudes were hardening. The police were able to count more than 500 teenage gangs, roaming the streets, looking for trouble. The gangs had wonderful, romantic-sounding names: the Rams, the Fanwoods, the Jesters, the Dragons, the Egyptian Kings. They didn't carry Uzis or AK-47s like the crack gangs do today. But the gang members of the late 1950s were tough, street-smart young men, guarding their turfs jealously, desperate to prove their manhood, ready to rumble in a minute.

These were the days that were glamorized in *West Side Story*.

But there was no singing or dancing at the Highbridge Pool on the night of July 30, 1957. There was no magic in the air, and there was no Maria. What happened that night was frighteningly real.

An ugly confrontation had been bubbling since the pool opened for the summer, right after Memorial Day. Highbridge Park sits on a bluff at the northern end of Manhattan, with splendid views of the Harlem River and the red-brick tenement houses of the South Bronx. Since Highbridge Park was owned by the city, anyone had a perfect legal right to play baseball there, or gaze off at the river or swim in the park's bigger-than-Olympic-size pool. For decades, however, the pool had been a place for white children. This wasn't written anywhere, but the black and Puerto Rican kids who lived in the neighborhoods to the south just didn't go swimming at Highbridge Park.

By 1957, those kinds of barriers were falling all over America. For the first time that summer, large numbers of black children were coming up from Harlem with their towels and swimsuits. Puerto Rican kids were coming too, from the East Harlem barrio.

The white, mostly Irish-American residents of Washington Heights were horrified. "An invasion," they called it, of "our pool."

The nastiness escalated as the summer wore on. Some of this played out in public. The usual racial slurs were tossed back and forth—"spic" and "mick" and "nigger" and those other hurtful words. More than once, the hard feelings erupted into fistfights in the blocks around the park.

Some of the ill will was more hidden. All over Washington Heights that summer, arguments were erupting at apartment dinner tables. It was the old story of us-against-them. You know the scenario. Here you are, in a white-Irish neighborhood. For the first time, these new people have started coming around. Your sister's at that boy-crazy age. One night, you come home for supper and you announce—half teasing, half mad—"Louise was at the pool, and she was making eyes at one of the Spanish boys, one of the

Spics." And then your mother says, "Louise, you stay away from those people."

Multiply that conversation by a few hundred or a few thousand. Before long, you're living in a pressure cooker. Some of it was almost unwitting, but the anger ran deep—touching the parents, the children, just about everyone. And it didn't take long for the members of the leading local youth gangs to get drawn into the growing hostility.

Three main gangs vied for power in this part of Manhattan. The Dragons were the Puerto Rican gang. Most of the Egyptian Kings were black. But the largest gang in New York that summer was the Jesters, working-class Irish kids who came from Washington Heights.

They had plenty to feud about.

In mid-June, the Jesters had challenged the Egyptian Kings to a stickball game, fifty cents a man. The Jesters won, but the Egyptian Kings accused them of cheating and refused to pay.

A few nights after that, a group of forty or so Egyptian Kings jumped five Jesters. No one was badly hurt, but whispers of revenge were being passed around the neighborhood. On Sunday, July 28, a Jester was stabbed by one of the Puerto Rican Dragons, whose members were sometimes aligned with the black gang. That turned the heat up another few degrees.

Feelings ran so high, in fact, that the leaders of the three gangs began exchanging private messages. They decided to make one final attempt to avert an all-out gang war.

July 30 was a humid Tuesday. A meeting was set for 10:30 P.M. at the main gate to the Highbridge Pool. Each of the three gangs was to send two representatives. All weapons were to be left at home. Everyone else was to stay away.

No one lived up to the agreement. Secretly, all three gangs had organized ambush parties. By ten o'clock, these other gang members were already hiding in the bushes and lingering in the shadows near the pool. They were well armed and ready to pounce.

Michael Farmer and Roger McShane were the official Jester representatives. (The Jesters' supreme leader decided wisely to sit this one out.) Farmer and McShane reached the steps of the pool a few minutes before ten thirty. The leaders of the other gangs were already waiting: Charles Horton and Leoncio DeLeon of the Egyptian Kings, Louis Alvarez and George Melendez of the Dragons. But the peace parley never took place.

Before Farmer and McShane made it up the steps, the night exploded in violence. The other gang members came rushing from the shadows, screaming, cursing, throwing punches, swinging knives and sticks. Horton pulled out a three-foot machete, which he dug right into Farmer's gut. As Farmer doubled over, a fourteen-year-old boy who was known as "Little King" plunged a knife so hard into Farmer's back it sunk all the way into the chest cavity.

"Thanks a lot," the boy said, as Farmer collapsed. He had always wanted to feel the sensation of metal cutting into bone, he explained later to a police detective.

McShane tried running, but he didn't get far. Louis Alvarez of the Dragons caught him in the chest with a second machete. McShane stumbled, bleeding, to the edge of the park.

"Find my friend," he shouted to a taxi driver who pulled up to the curb. "Find my friend."

The cabbie wasn't sure what McShane was talking about. But he could see the boy was bleeding hard. So he loaded him into the taxi and drove to Columbia-Presbyterian Hospital. The emergency-room doctors saved McShane's life. But by the time police reached the park and found where his friend had fallen, Farmer had already lost a tremendous amount of blood. He died before the ambulance could reach Cabrini Hospital.

The police responded in droves that night. They swept teenagers off the street all over upper Manhattan. The interrogations went on into the morning. The cops wanted everyone who was in the park that night.

The story hit the papers with the force of Horton's machete swing, although the details got twisted a little in the telling. Farmer wasn't quite the little angel the papers made him out to be. He was, after all, a top leader of the city's biggest youth gang. And although he had suffered from a mild case of polio as a child, Farmer was absolutely not the "crippled boy" the front-page articles described. He had recovered fully from the polio and was an outstanding high school athlete.

Nonetheless, his death was an awful, unjustifiable crime. Not surprisingly, it created an instant public furor. The sheer brutality of the melee was bad enough. The racial element made it even worse. By the time the police round-ups were over, forty teenagers were in custody.

Thirty-three of them were younger than the age of fifteen. They were marched off to the Warwick State Training School and similar institutions, where most of them received thorough prepschool educations in the ways of violent crime.

The seven others—the so-called adults, who had reached their fifteenth birthdays—had even bigger problems on their hands. Under New York law, they were eligible for a full measure of the state's judicial system. The charge against them was premeditated murder. The maximum possible penalty: a one-way trip to the death house at Sing Sing.

I didn't know much about drug abuse back then. What little I knew about gang warfare I had learned from reading the newspapers. I was born in 1924 and grew up the third of four children—the older of two boys—in a fairly secure Irish-Catholic family in Tuckahoe, a tiny town about an hour north of New York City. My father was a vice-president at National City Bank. My mother stayed at home. I was one of those Catholic boys who always wanted to be a priest. In my case, the urge struck for the first time when I was in fourth grade. A young, dynamic Sister Reginald had outlined life's options for me (adding, no doubt, an extra measure of luster to her description of the priestly vocation). I already had the idea that I wanted to help people. I never really considered doing anything else. I went into the seminary prep at fourteen. I was ordained at twenty-six, in 1951. I spent most of the next few years as a parish priest in the tiny Hudson River towns of Ardsley and Walden, organizing altar boys and running CYO basketball tournaments. Then, unexpectedly, Cardinal Spellman transferred me to St. Patrick's Cathedral, the grand seat of the Archdiocese of New York, the most famous church in America.

St. Pat's, with its spires rising over Fifth Avenue, can be an awe-inspiring place—and a powerful symbol for the majesty of the Roman Catholic church. But for a young priest, it's not necessarily the greatest place to be assigned. The cathedral is not like a normal parish. There's little sense of community. And the place is so laden with church bureaucracy, it's a wonder anything ever gets done there. Priests in New York used to have a saying: "The cathedral is a nice place to have been." The thought didn't need to be completed out loud: not such a nice place to be.

But something was always happening at the cathedral. People would drop by at all hours, asking for help or just wanting to talk to a priest. The priests on staff would take turns on "first duty." That meant you were the one to speak with whomever happened to appear at the rectory door. Often, these were people who, for one reason or another, hadn't gotten satisfaction in their home parishes. So they'd come down to headquarters, which is how they thought of the cathedral.

One night early in August of 1957, I got a call in my room from the switchboard operator. She said a woman was downstairs, asking for a priest. There are five small parlors on the main floor of the cathedral rectory, and this woman was waiting for me in one of them.

I came down and introduced myself to a plain-looking, middle-aged woman. She was obviously distraught. Her face was pale as an altarcloth. Her eyes were clearly bloodshot. You could see that she'd been crying. Her voice trembled a little as she began to speak.

She said her name was Mrs. McCarthy, and she lived in St. Catherine of Genoa parish, up in Washington Heights. I knew the church. It was on Riverside Drive at 152d Street. My mother and father were married there. The area used to be quite elegant. But over the years the demographics had shifted. By the late 1950s, it was basically a sagging neighborhood of rundown tenements and old brownstones that had been chopped into apartments. The pastor who had been assigned there in the *bon ton* days was still there. But his reaction to the changing community had been to build a fence around the church. Mrs. McCarthy said she had been over to see him. But he told her he didn't think there was much he could do.

Then, she told me a story that would change my life.

Her son Johnny, she said, was one of the boys arrested for the Farmer murder. The judge had sent Johnny over to the prison ward at Bellevue Hospital for a battery of psychiatric tests. Mrs. McCarthy said she had been raising the boy alone. Her husband, a severe alcoholic, had died when Johnny was ten. The family was now on welfare, and they lived in a ratty apartment building on 152d Street. Charles Horton, the number-two man in the Egyptian Kings, the one who swung the machete at Michael Farmer, lived directly across the hall. "Big Man," as Horton was known around the neighborhood, used and sold heroin, Mrs. McCarthy said, and Johnny was scared to death of Big Man. Alternating threats and ego-massage, Big Man used to get Johnny to run menial errands for the gang— and to come out when they needed an extra body. Johnny was the only white face in that tough black gang.

Her son was with the Egyptian Kings the night Michael Farmer was killed, Mrs. McCarthy said. But first-degree murder? That just didn't sound like her soft-spoken son. Was there any way I could help?

Now, I had no idea what I could do for Mrs. McCarthy. And for all I knew, precious Johnny McCarthy was a cold-blooded killer. But I had never been the kind of priest who could easily brush people off. I was compulsive that way. Plenty of times, I had been taken in by the people who came to the cathedral with terrible tales of woe—only some of which turned out to be true. New York's expert con-artists have all discovered St. Patrick's Cathedral. Still, I would tell myself, that's just the cost of doing business as a priest.

After hearing a little more of Mrs. McCarthy's story, I told the priest on second duty, "Hey, cover for me for a little while." Then, this woman and I climbed into a cab, and we rode down to Bellevue.

When we got up to the hospital's prison ward, out came this frail, little baby-faced boy. He had wispy reddish hair and these huge, sad eyes. He did not look much like a murderer to me. He sounded mildly retarded. When he and I sat down at a table and began talking, he seemed to have the mind of about a seven-year-old. He was also a grand-mal epileptic, who suffered periodic seizures. His fifteenth birthday had arrived just two days before Michael Farmer was killed, a terrible coincidence. That's what qualified him for a seat in Sing Sing's electric chair.

I spent three hours talking with the boy before I left Bellevue. He told me Big Man had made him come along that night and had given him some pills to take before they left 152d Street. There's no denying he was in the park that night, Johnny said. But he swore he'd never hit Farmer or McShane.

When I finally got back to the cathedral, the questions were still racing through my head: What was such a pathetic kid doing in the middle of something as awful as this? How could teenage street fighting have turned so grotesquely violent? What made young people so eager to kill each other? Where had their consciences gone? What could the church do? What could the city do? What could anyone do to stop this carnage?

Over the months that followed, I suppose you could say I became obsessed with the Farmer case. I went to the police department and got the names of the other young people who were arrested. I went around and interviewed every last one of them—at Warwick State, or Bellevue, or the Brooklyn House of Detention, where most of the older boys were being held.

They told amazing stories, each more pathetic than the one that preceded it. They spoke of poverty and boredom and broken homes. They described the excitement and comradeship of the gangs. Inevitably, after we had talked for a while, the kid would burst into tears and before long I'd be pulling out my handkerchief, too.

One other common denominator ran through all these unfortunate stories, and I ultimately became convinced it was at the very center of what was wrong.

Drugs.

The gang members in the late 1950s had gotten heavily into drugs. Heroin, mostly. They were using and selling. Many of them were addicted. This had not yet received much public attention, but it had become an important fact of life. The gang members were also taking pills called cibas, Ciba Doriden, which gave them such splitting headaches that they needed a few shots of Cosanyl cough syrup to make the headaches go away.

Drugs had lifted the art of urban street fighting to an entirely new level of viciousness. Much of the gangs' warfare was over who could sell drugs where, and a good deal of the bravery they brought into battle came from the needles they were jamming into their arms and the pills they were dropping down their throats. This was certainly true the night Michael Farmer was killed. Many of the boys who came at him were stoned out of their minds. Big Man Horton— and I came ultimately to believe that he was the most sinned against of them all—was so wasted he couldn't even remember what had happened in the park.

The trial opened on January 10 in Manhattan Supreme Court. All seven of the so-called adults were tried together, with a total of twenty-seven lawyers defending them.

I was in court just about every day. The assistant district attorney delighted in all the gang slang and the funny-sounding nicknames, which he repeated over and over again. He told the jury that Michael

Farmer's death was premeditated murder, orchestrated by Leroy "the Magician" Birch, the Egyptian Kings' seventeen-year-old "warlord." "Big Man" Horton, the prosecutor said, was the one with the machete, and Louis "Little Jesse" Alvarez, another seventeen-year-old, had a knife. Leoncio DeLeon, known on the street as "Jello," swung a wooden club, the prosecutor said. The three other "adult" brawlers, the prosecutor charged, were Richard Hills, George Melendez, and Johnny McCarthy.

The prosecution and the defense fought bitterly over the introduction of the autopsy report, which called a deep stab wound to Farmer's back the primary cause of death.

The defense lawyers did what they could to protect their clients. One portrayed Farmer's death as an "unfortunate accident." Another lawyer put the blame on "racial tensions in our city" and on the detective who "brainwashed and bludgeoned" his client into confessing.

The trial went on like this for ninety-six acrimonious days, a total of 1.5 million words, enough to fill 6,000 pages of transcript. When the jury finally came back on April 15, the foreman announced a split decision: Horton and Alvarez guilty of second-degree murder; Birch and DeLeon guilty of second-degree manslaughter; McCarthy, Hills, and Melendez acquitted on all counts.

The trial had been a showcase for an important, evolving social change that no one was interested in dealing with. Michael Farmer's death was, in a very real sense, the end of old-fashioned gang warfare in New York, the end of *West Side Story*. The gangs had become so violent—and the gang members so stoned all the time—that the street-corner rumble had lost much of its allure.

At the same time, a new era of urban history was dawning. We were at the beginning of the modern hostility among the races. We were at the beginning of something else, too. The Farmer case was the opening chapter in America's modern age of drug abuse.

To me, the next step seemed clear: government and the church had to find some way to get involved. I didn't have any idea how.

Not back then, at least. I was just a thirty-three-year-old priest. I had no influence at all over the politicians who ran New York. I didn't have a whole lot more influence over the leaders of the Catholic church.

But I was a priest, and that meant something. Priests are supposed to act. I knew in my gut that somehow I was going to be part of that action. It took me several more years to figure out where the answers might lie. But I got right on with the search.

A CENTURY
OF FRUSTRATION 3

Health is much too serious a matter to be left entirely to Doctors, Psychiatrists, Psychologists, and the established Medical System.

—Georges Clemenceau, premier of France during World War I

I began studying America's sporadic attempts over the years to confront the problem of drug abuse. Few stories are as depressing as this one.

The cycle of disappointment goes all the way back to the early 1850s, when drug addiction was first declared a threat to the public welfare.

Opium was the problem drug back then.

Most of the addicts, it turned out, were women who started taking the opium to ward off the cramps and depression that came with their menstrual periods. The drug was legal. It was cheap and widely available. It sold for a few pennies a dose at corner groceries and candy stores.

But there's this thing called tolerance, and no one had accounted for that. The nineteenth-century opium users built up a quick tolerance to their magic menstrual medication. After just a few uses, these women needed stronger and stronger doses to deliver the same kind of relief. Before long, they were craving opium at other times of the month and acquiring full-fledged addictions.

It wasn't a pretty sight. These respectable women were stumbling around their kitchens and living rooms, blasted out of their minds. Dinner wasn't getting cooked. The clothes weren't getting washed. The children weren't getting off to school. All the other things that women of that day were expected to do weren't getting done. This created tension in their families and left the women feeling even more depressed—and even more eager for the temporary euphoria that the opium brought.

By today's standards, the total number of opium addicts was relatively small. But the alarm was taken seriously enough that in 1853, the U.S. Public Health Service stepped in, declaring a public health emergency. Opium was placed under strict legal controls. The drug was yanked off the candy-store shelves. Not surprisingly, a black market grew up. And many American women kept using opium until, some years later, the drug just seemed to run its natural course and fade from popularity.

All the while though, no one had bothered to focus much attention on the women who now had no legal means to answer their addictions. And no one gave much thought to the medical problem of premenstrual syndrome, which had driven the women toward the drug in the first place.

It's a pattern that's been repeated so many times since then they are almost impossible to count.

In the years that immediately followed the nation's first drug crisis, America fought three wars, one for each generation. Every time, the wounded came home heavily sedated on some different drug, and a new generation of addicts was promptly dumped onto society. After the Civil War, the soldiers were pumped up with opium, on doctors' orders. By the time the Spanish-American War came around, doctors knew about the dangers of opium addiction, so they turned instead to opium's child, morphine. It was a good painkiller, but morphine turned out to be even more addictive than opium. The same thing happened in World War I: Morphine was considered too addictive, so the medical profession turned to a new wonder drug, the child of morphine, heroin.

All this time, the problem of drug addiction was left mostly in the hands of medicine. Physicians owned the body, and doctors figured they could cure addiction as they'd cured so many other ills. Addicts were sent onto hospital wards, where they lay around on clean sheets, waiting for the medical magic. The men in white coats came by every now and then, dispensing medication and never asking the patients to take any responsibility for their own recoveries. Whenever a patient created a scene, the doctors were standing by, ready with another injection of sedatives. The addicts loved it.

About all this accomplished was to fill up the veterans' hospitals with drug addicts. Almost no one was ever cured, and by the late 1920s medicine was pretty much discredited as the answer to drug addiction.

Society turned next to the criminal-justice system. What doctors and nurses couldn't do, locked doors and steel bars would. Drug laws were toughened. Huge prison sentences were handed out. But again, few addicts beat their addictions in jail. In some cases, the prison walls succeeded in separating addicts from their drugs, temporarily. But drugs often found their way onto the cellblocks, and the threat of prison seemed to scare almost nobody from using drugs on the outside. And, of course, the minute the prison gates swung open, inmates would go right back to the drugs that got them locked up in the first place.

With World War II, the cycle of failure rolled on. The wounded came from Europe and Asia. This time, a synthetic narcotic, methadone, was added to the rainbow of painkillers. Yet another generation of drug addicts was put onto the street.

The medical establishment stepped forward with still another highly touted "cure." These were called detoxification centers. They were set up in hospitals across America. Generally, the addicts were more than happy to check in, especially when they were broke or feeling burned out. They received nourishing food, time to relax, a little coddling and few demands. The clean sheets and the gentle surroundings were terrific. But few of the addicts stuck around for the full twenty-one days. Most of them were gone after a week or so. That was long enough to flush the impurities from the bloodstream and head back to the street with a much-reduced tolerance for drugs.

Typically, the addicts returned to the needle the day they left the hospital. Some didn't even wait that long. In one program at New York's Manhattan General Hospital, a windowsill lifeline kept the detox patients fully supplied. They hung strings from their windows. A five-dollar bill tied to the end would be exchanged on the sidewalk for a glassine envelope of heroin.

The government money kept flowing. But by the early 1950s, it was generally conceded that both medicine and prison had failed to do much about drug addiction—except possibly make the problem worse.

So a new candidate was drafted, psychiatry. State mental hospitals opened new wings to treat drug addicts. The addicts checked in and stayed drugged up for most of their stay. Private psychiatric hospitals opened their own programs—offering plusher surroundings—for addicts with money or generous insurance plans. But the psychiatrists had no more success than the physicians or the wardens. In New York City, the most monumental experiment in drug treatment up to that time opened at Riverside Hospital. In one year, $8 million was spent. Two psychiatrists were assigned to every addict. Not a single addict was turned around.

Various other blips appeared on the drug-treatment landscape: Christian fundamentalism, acupuncture, Buddhism, miracle drugs of one variety or another. All of it got fawning media attention. None of it made much of a dent. At one point, the federal government even opened two huge facilities that were part hospital, part prison. One was in Lexington, Kentucky, the other in Fort Worth, Texas. New York State set up a program on the same model, called Article IX, on Ward's Island in the middle of the East River.

Give these programs credit for trying to blend more than one approach to treatment. But still, they could never figure out precisely how to get the addicts to stay off drugs.

And that, essentially, is where the science of drug treatment sat in the summer of 1957, when Michael Farmer was killed and I wandered half blindly into the subject of drug abuse. Almost every discipline had taken its crack at the problem. Nothing was working. And we had already lost a tremendous amount of time.

Soon after the Farmer trial, Cardinal Spellman transferred me from the cathedral to Our Lady of the Assumption, a huge parish in the Pelham Bay section of the Bronx. The area, which had once been largely Irish, was growing more and more Italian. Economically, it was a step or two better off than the Washington Heights of Michael Farmer and his friends. But the problems, I discovered, weren't really so different. Drugs got to Pelham Bay before I did, and they had made themselves at home.

Assumption had all the programs and activities you'd expect from a good Catholic parish of its day. We had a parochial school and an altar society and a Knights of Columbus chapter and Saturday morning religious instruction for the kids who went to public school. We had a big crew of altar boys and a gigantic CYO sports program.

But most of these efforts, it seemed to me, were designed to save the saved. And I was growing increasingly concerned about the kids who were standing in the shadows, the ones who didn't even think they needed to be saved. Monsignor John Kenney, the pastor, was trying to build a strong parish. Naturally, he was concerned that I not spend too much time and energy working with these troubled kids from "outside the parish," which is what just about everyone at Assumption thought drug users were.

The monsignor was a dynamic and decent man. His generation just didn't understand what we were up against as the 1950s drew to a close. Pelham Bay was drowning from the drug problem, and all the community wanted to do was deny. The attitude at Our Lady of the Assumption was that the drug addicts were all from St. Theresa's Parish across the way. This wasn't true, of course. One young man died of a heroin overdose practically right across the street from the Assumption rectory. And the biggest drug-copping area in all of the North Bronx was in our own backyard in Throgs Neck, at the corner of Morris and Tremont avenues.

I started talking about drugs in my sermons. I held some discussion groups over at the parish house. I began getting calls from parents, people in the parish, saying, "My boy just got arrested for the third time. He's a good kid, but I think it's the drugs." Or, "My daughter doesn't want to do anything anymore. She just sits in her room, staring into space. Now she's stealing money from my purse, and we just found a hypodermic needle taped underneath the sink in the bathroom."

More and more, it was becoming obvious that we had a social problem of major proportions on our hands. I still didn't know what to do about it. I paid calls on anyone I could think of—psychiatrists, social workers, the welfare and public-health people, the police and the local school officials. They were all very nice. But it turned out none of them had a clue about what to do, either.

All I knew was that more and more parents were calling. More and more kids were showing up at the rectory door. Drugs seemed to be growing more prevalent. It wasn't until the summer of 1959 that I began hearing talk about a place in Westport, Connecticut, a rambling old white house where amazing things were supposedly happening. The place was called Synanon, and it was the East Coast outpost of a small program that had sprung up in California.

Early one Saturday morning, I drove up to Westport, an affluent suburban town on the north side of Long Island Sound. I eventually found my way to the house I was looking for on Green Farms Road. I parked my car. As I was getting out, another car pulled up beside mine. A short, balding man climbed out.

He was an intense gentleman, full of nervous energy. He introduced himself as we walked together up to the door. He said his name was Dan Casriel, and he was a psychiatrist in New York. He was up to check out Synanon, too.

The name sounded familiar, but I couldn't place it at first.

"Casriel, Casriel," I said. "Didn't I just read an article by you in the *Herald-Tribune*? Do you believe what you said?"

The week before, Casriel had written a series of articles on drug addiction. He had studied the problem for many years, and it had left him extremely pessimistic.

With addicts, he concluded, there are really only two things you can do: put them on an island with sharks in the water and leave them there forever; or give them all the drugs they want and get out of their way. Society has no other options, he wrote.

"Of course, I believe it," Casriel said as we reached the front door.

The two of us walked into that house together at about 9:30 in the morning. What we saw and heard inside left us speechless. We were destroyed, both of us. We couldn't believe it.

The place was filled with drug addicts. Big-time, serious drug addicts. Heroin junkies and pillheads. People who had been addicted for ten—in some cases twenty—years. People who had expected to use hard drugs until it killed them.

And here they were, pouring their hearts out, talking about how they were turning their lives around. They had invested everything they had in their treatment. They had emptied their pockets and put all their possessions in a pile on the center of the floor. That way, their lives would be their most important treasures.

A houseful of junkies, living together. Without violence. Without doctors. Without guards. For people like Casriel and me, this was nothing short of amazing. These drug addicts had made powerful commitments to a new family, one that would challenge and support them as they battled to reclaim their lives from drugs.

The process wasn't easy, the director of the Westport house, David Deitch, assured us. It demanded a rugged honesty. The residents had to strip themselves bare and rebuild their entire value systems. But with enough commitment, the director said, it could be done.

Casriel and I sat there, our jaws open and our eyes wide. We couldn't leave. I was supposed to hear confessions back in the Bronx that afternoon, but I remained at Westport through the night, spellbound. I got back home just in time for early morning Mass. When I left, Casriel was still at the Synanon house, tears running down his cheeks.

ENTERING THE FRAY 4

> *The worst sin toward our fellow creatures is not to hate them but to be indifferent to them, that's the essence of inhumanity.*
>
> —George Bernard Shaw

For me, Synanon was a godsend. Finally, I had somewhere to direct those kids whose lives were being ruined by drugs. Over the next three years, I became one of Synanon's biggest boosters.

The group's founder, Chuck Dederich, had discovered something that all those doctors and criminologists and social workers hadn't figured out after treating drug addicts for 100 years. The drug is not the addict's fundamental problem. The real problem is a complicated mix of factors inside the addict's mind. These factors are psychosocial, theological, and sexual—and uniformly hard to reach. The only way to cure addiction, the Synanon founder knew, was to rebuild the addict's entire system of values.

Dederich had no professional training in the treatment of drug abuse. He had grown up in Ohio, in a middle-class Catholic family. Although he was a voracious reader, he dropped out of Notre Dame, got married, and went to work. He had obvious smarts and a rough-edged charisma, and he rose easily into the executive ranks of the Gulf Oil Company.

He also happened to be a falling-down drunk. His heavy drinking eventually cost him the job at Gulf and several others. It cost him two marriages, as well. In 1957, he was out of work again, living in a furnished room near the beach in Santa Monica, California, and finally ready to make a change.

He began attending meetings of Alcoholics Anonymous. But

quickly, he decided that AA's twelve-step sobriety program was just not intense enough for him. So one day, he cashed a thirty-three-dollar unemployment check, rented a shabby storefront in nearby Ocean Park, and started conducting his own meetings.

Dederich was a terrifically engaging speaker. He had read Emerson and Thoreau and Lao-tzu at Notre Dame. He could quote them eloquently and weave their insights—with a heavy sprinkling of Freud's—into his long, heartfelt talks.

In the early days, he called his group the TLC Club, for Tender Loving Care. But there was nothing tender about Dederich's manner. He was loud. He was profane. He would speak with brutal honesty about how he had wrecked his life and the lives of those who loved him. He demanded the same frank admissions from the people who showed up. He insisted that they confront each other—frankly, aggressively—over even the smallest dishonesties. Everything was to be brought into the open.

People began flocking to Dederich's supercharged meetings, and not just alcoholics. Drug addicts started coming too. The meetings would often go late into the evening. The participants could be heard crying, screaming at each other, and confessing the most intimate personal failings. These confrontation sessions usually ended on a note of mutual support. And the people would head off into the night, invigorated. Dederich called the meetings symposiums, or seminars—until a confused junkie one night mushed the two words together. That's where the name Synanon came from.

Dederich was off and running. He rented an old warehouse at the beach to handle the overflow crowd. His celebrity spread across the country. He was profiled in national magazines and on network television. Liberal Californians made big donations. Steve Allen sang his praises on *The Tonight Show*. By 1962, just four years after he started Synanon, Connecticut's Thomas Dodd stood on the floor of the U.S. Senate, describing "a man-made miracle" on the California beachfront. Said Dodd: "Addicts for the first time are reclaiming their lives."

A few years later, Chuck Dederich and Synanon would go off the deep end. They would become a crazed, violent cult—just one step this side of Jim Jones. They would arm themselves to the teeth and organize their own militia. They would attack their so-called enemies and leave a rattlesnake in the mailbox of an unfriendly lawyer. Dederich himself would grow paranoid and start drinking again, losing any grip on reality.

But despite this depressing end, Dederich had some brilliant insights about the treatment of drug addiction. Thirty years ago, the world benefited from those insights. It benefits from them today.

While Dederich was building his organization in California, the people of Our Lady of the Assumption parish in the Bronx were growing increasingly worried about drugs. Crime was becoming a constant part of city life. And the criminals weren't all coming into the neighborhood from the black and Hispanic sections to the south, as most of the parishioners wanted to believe. Often, the criminals were the sons and sometimes even the daughters of Pelham Bay, hunting money for drugs. We set up an organization called SOS, Supporters of Synanon. We held huge fund-raising dinners, putting three thousand people a night in the Chateau Pelham, the biggest banquet hall in that part of the Bronx.

New York had more drug addicts than anywhere else in America. By far. Yet Synanon was still basically a West Coast operation. No real treatment went on at the house in Westport. It was essentially a recruitment and induction center. So we channeled dozens— eventually hundreds—of New York City addicts through Westport and out to California.

We worked with the police and the welfare workers to get people into Synanon. Some of the kids were thrilled to learn real treatment was available. Others had to be pushed. We came up with a system. We'd say to one of the detectives, "Bobby over there is driving his family crazy. He's dealing drugs, and he's stoned out of his head."

And the detective would say, "Okay, what's the address?"

I would talk to the mother and father and tell them, "Hey, your son is breaking your heart. You don't know what to do. Tomorrow morning, the police will be coming over to the house around two o'clock. They will tell Bobby they are ready to arrest him. A great sense of urgency will be created, and then the cops will say, 'Well, we'll give you one more chance, bring you over to Father O'Brien.' "

They would wheel the kid over to me, and I'd run him up to Westport.

I was in my glory. I always felt religion was about "resurrection." Wasn't that the central role of the priest—an instrument for helping people revive their lives? I had a place to send these kids. I could intervene. I could motivate them. And if they were not so motivated, the police and the social workers would help. I was in touch all the time with Chuck Dederich's people out in California, and with David Deitch, the director of the Westport house. I also stayed in contact with Dan Casriel, the psychiatrist I'd met that first day in the driveway. He remained extremely interested.

At last, I felt, we were doing something positive about drugs.

It turned out that Casriel and I weren't the only people in New York who had stumbled across Synanon. Through a very different course, the Brooklyn office of the New York State Department of Probation ended up in much the same place we were.

The chief probation officer in Brooklyn back then was a small, somber man named Joseph Shelly. He was miles from the stereotypical half-a-cop probation officer. Shelly dressed more like an undertaker, and he had social-work degrees from Fordham and the University of Chicago. He would sit for hours in his back office, poring over academic journals. Then, he would experiment with the things he had read about. He created a special probation caseload for teenage offenders and one for probationers who had severe psychiatric problems. He set up the office's first statistical record-keeping system and even hired two doctoral students from New York University to run a group-therapy clinic for people on probation.

These things are all common practice today. But back then, Shelly's office was on the cutting edge of innovative criminology. One of the probation department's biggest problems—then as now—was the large number of drug addicts on the client list. They made terrible probationers. They were constantly getting rearrested and ruining Shelly's precious success statistics.

"We hoped we would be able to show, year by year, we were reducing the percentage of failures and the amount of crime," said Alexander Bassin, one of the doctoral students, who became Shelly's research and education director. "The figures didn't back us up." And those recalcitrant heroin addicts were to blame.

One day early in 1963, Bassin was called into the boss's office. Shelly said he had been reading a not-so-highly-regarded academic journal, *Reader's Digest*. He came across an article by a police lieutenant from Oakland, California, touting the benefits of something called Nalline.

These were the days before widespread drug testing—and before courts clamped down on police search-and-seizure practices. The lieutenant's name was Charles Brown. According to the article, Nalline could be injected into the arm of a suspected drug user. If drugs were present in the bloodstream, the Nalline would turn brown. "Part of my job at the time was to go around to probationers and say, 'Are you using,'" Bassin said. "And then I'd have to determine if the pimples on the inside of their arms were real pinpricks or just mosquito bites."

This Nalline might be a better way. So Bassin sent off a letter to the National Institute of Mental Health outside Washington, asking for money to set up a Nalline lab at the Brooklyn probation office.

Within days, Dr. Carl Anderson, a drug- and alcohol-abuse consultant with the institute, was on the phone. He told Shelly and Bassin to come on down.

"We don't share *Reader's Digest*'s enthusiasm," Anderson told his visitors right after they arrived at the institute's headquarters. Nalline was nothing but hype, he said. The test results can't be believed. The drug can be administered safely only by a physician. And if a drug user had recently injected heroin, an injection of Nalline could be fatal.

This left Shelly and Bassin a little puzzled. Why had Anderson dragged them down to Maryland to tell them that? But Anderson had something else in mind—two other things, in fact.

Would the Brooklyn probation office be interested in testing a more promising drug-detection method, something called thin-layer chromatography? Anderson wanted to know. It was a urine test used until then only on racehorses.

Sure, they said. But that wasn't the main thing on Anderson's mind.

"Halfway house," he said, just like that.

Today, that expression is well known: a place somewhere between freedom and incarceration. But in early 1963, the concept was just being hashed out in Shelly's academic journals.

"There's maybe half a dozen of them in the entire country," Anderson told the two men. "We'd like you to go out and see what they're doing. Maybe this is something that could be used with drug addicts."

It's worth a try, Bassin and Shelly agreed. They would move ahead, they told Anderson, assuming the feds will pay.

The money will be there, Anderson promised.

Quickly, Bassin and Shelly arranged a cross-country tour of drug-testing labs and halfway houses. The two of them would go, of course. But Anderson had suggested they also bring along a criminologist and a psychiatrist. So Bassin called two of his friends. One of them was Herbert Bloch, a criminology professor at Brooklyn College. The other was Dan Casriel, the Manhattan psychiatrist who had discovered Synanon the same day I had.

The four of them made several stops before they got to Santa

Monica. They met with the scientist who had invented thin-layer chromatography. His testing system certainly sounded promising. They paid a call on Lieutenant Brown at the Oakland Police Department. The visitors found him less impressive in person than he had sounded in the pages of *Reader's Digest*, just as Anderson had said.

By the time the group reached Synanon, Casriel needed no convincing at all. It took the other three about five minutes to decide: This was the model for their new halfway house. Here was a group of addicts, living together, committed to absolute honesty, getting along entirely without drugs. The beachfront warehouse was immaculately clean. The residents were polite as altar boys. Casriel immediately ran into several addicts he had treated back at Metropolitan Hospital in New York. Except they were no longer the scrawny, bleary-eyed people he remembered. Now, they looked healthy and fit and more upbeat than he had ever seen them.

Chuck Dederich was a tremendously engaging leader and an odd man. He spoke in a gruff tone, and his sentences had a way of running on and on.

"We attempt to create an extended family of the type found in preliterate tribes, with a strong, perhaps autocratic father figure, who dispenses firm justice combined with warm concern, who is a model extolling inner-directed convictions about the old-fashioned virtues of honesty, sobriety, learning and hard work." That's how Dederich spoke. But somehow, his words were mesmerizing.

The visitors weren't quite sure what it all meant. But the results looked encouraging, indeed.

Shelly broached the idea of Dederich's helping to start a Synanon-like program in New York.

He said he might be interested—but only if all the money would be turned over to him and no one would ever question how a single penny was spent.

That sent shivers down Joe Shelly's bureaucratic spine. He could just imagine selling that one to the federal government. The idea was not pursued again.

Nevertheless, as the travelers prepared to leave California, they knew they had the concept they were looking for—if not the man to run it. In the end, Casriel decided to linger in California after the others left for New York. He stayed at Synanon for several months and wrote a favorable book about the experience: *So Fair a House*.

The other three returned to New York.

Bassin got busy on the formal grant application. Shelly started looking at real estate.

On April 15, a letter arrived from Maryland. Grant No. 1292 had been approved, $390,000. It was enough to run a drug lab and a twenty-five-bed halfway house for five years.

Through a realtor, Shelly found a vacant mansion in the New York City borough of Staten Island, about two miles from the town of Tottenville. It was built as a private residence by a man named Butler, but more recently had been a retirement home for merchant seamen. It had twenty-five rooms and beautiful views of Raritan Bay. Most important of all, the owner, John Minirvini, would rent to Shelly for $833 a month.

Shelly signed a one-year lease and began planning for a September 1 opening. But as the day grew nearer, this new program didn't have a director and it didn't have a name.

Bassin went to the only place he could think of for assistance, the New York headquarters of Alcoholics Anonymous. Dederich had come out of AA, after all. It seemed like as good a place to look as any.

After several candidates said, "No thank you," the people at AA sent over a former shoe salesman named Dean Colcord. He didn't have any training in the treatment of drug addicts. But then, neither had Dederich. Colcord was also a longtime alcoholic. And he was willing to take the job.

So he was hired.

Shelly tried to organize a naming contest in the probation department office. Various suggestions were kicked around. No one was too happy with any of them. Finally, Bassin dreamed up the one that stuck. Riding to work one day on the subway, he tried scribbling various word combinations on a yellow legal pad until he found one that sounded right.

Drug Addicts Treated on Probation. D-A-Y-T-O-P. The Y got inserted because it made the acronym easier to pronounce.

"At the time, various psychiatric programs, trying to get away from an institutional idea, were calling themselves Lodge," Bassin remembered. "That sounded good to my ear. So I suggested Daytop Lodge. No one could think of anything better. So that's what it was."

THE FINEST
OF INTENTIONS 5

Civilizations are the product or result of challenge and response; and they rise or fall, live or die with their ability or inability to respond properly and adequately to challenges.

—Arnold Toynbee, *A Study of History*

The doors to Daytop Lodge opened quietly on September 1, 1963.

For two weeks, there was no one around the old Butler Manor but Dean Colcord, his wife, Linda, and Topper, their dog. Bassin and Shelly were back at their office in downtown Brooklyn, trying to pull together a roster of twenty-five suitable probationers. They were looking for drug addicts with no history of violence or sexual crimes who had expressed at least some interest in getting off drugs.

The first recruit arrived September 16.

Charlie Devlin was a twenty-two-year-old heroin addict from Brooklyn. He was a short, stocky construction worker who had been using drugs since his early teens. He had just been arrested for possession of a hypodermic needle and a stolen television set. He talked tough, but he was obviously sharp, and he struck Bassin as relatively energetic for a junkie.

Devlin pleaded guilty to the possession charges, and the judge offered him a choice: a year at Rikers Island or a year in this new program that the probation department was setting up.

"I had just spent a few months in jail," Devlin recalled. "I knew jail. It had to be better than that. And I guess somewhere inside of me I always had that motivation of wanting to stop using drugs. It was really ruining my life." He took the deal.

The judge told him that two gentlemen were waiting for him at the probation office. "I was given directions and just told to go over," Devlin remembered. "No handcuffs, nobody escorting me. I guess the idea was to show some sort of trust." When he got to probation, Devlin was ushered inside and introduced to Bassin and Shelly.

"They made this big commotion over me," Devlin said. "'Oh, congratulations.' It was like I'd won a prize. You know, 'You've been selected, we know you can do it.' I got a real pep talk. But I still didn't really know what I was supposed to do."

Bassin gave him a token for the subway, a nickel for the Staten Island ferry and enough change to catch the train out to Tottenville. A couple of hours later, Dean Colcord met Devlin at the station. He was just as exuberant as Bassin and Shelly had been. "He was saying, 'Congratulations,' making a big to-do," Devlin said. "Then, he drove me out to this big house, overlooking Raritan Bay. Beautiful mansion. Big rolling hill outside. You could look out the windows and see the water. There were some houses, some nice middle-class houses, around it. Dean took me inside, and he said, 'You're the first one, and we expect a lot from you.' Then, he and his wife showed me this beautiful room, this big, spacious room. They told me, 'You can have any room you want.' Big, private showers. Now, I always lived in apartments, lower-income apartments. Never had anything this nice. But why not? Why not give it a chance? It was very nice. This was the farthest thing from jail. They were acting like I'd won the lottery or something."

Not much happened for the next couple of weeks. Devlin got friendly with the Colcords. He helped them get the house in order for the other probationers who were supposed to be coming soon. The Colcords took him along to the AA meetings they were still attending. But no real drug treatment was going on.

Finally, other residents began arriving. Number two was Bobby Byrd, a smooth-talking ex-con from Brownsville. Others trickled in. Among the first wave were John Ruocco, a beefy Italian kid from

Coney Island, and seventeen-year-old Bobby Boriello, who got in because a sympathetic judge was willing to overlook the minimum-age rule.

All the new residents came to the Lodge the same way: as an alternative to jail, compliments of the Brooklyn Probation Department. They didn't all know each other before Daytop. But they ran in similar circles. And most of them had friends in common or at least had done business with the same drug dealers.

As the bedrooms began filling up, Dean Colcord tried to put a program into place. Chuck Dederich had reluctantly allowed him to come out to Synanon for three weeks in August, and he had picked up a few tricks out there. He began calling house meetings in the morning, conducting seminars on sobriety in the afternoon and holding group-encounter sessions at night. These were all Synanon staples. Colcord had learned a few phrases out in California, too. He used them frequently: "That flips my gut," he would say when he was angry. Or he would ask the residents to "cop," or own up, to some transgression. Dan Casriel would stop by once a week to lead one of the discussion groups and give advice.

Still, the place had none of the intensity of Synanon. But by mid-October, some semblance of drug treatment was finally under way.

That was just about the time people in the neighborhood began figuring out that something peculiar was going on over at the old Butler mansion.

Brief stories had appeared in the newspapers back in April about the Brooklyn Probation Department's $390,000 grant. No one on Staten Island had paid much attention. And when John Minirvini agreed to lease his empty mansion for this new drug program, he knew better than to send out a press release. Nonetheless, by October the neighbors couldn't help wondering about the pale young men in white tee shirts who were out in the yard every afternoon, pulling weeds and planting shrubbery.

Word spread swiftly.

"Drug addicts."

"Sent to the mansion instead of jail."

"Twenty-five of them, moving into the neighborhood."

Now, there are probably not many communities in America—particularly back in 1963—where this would be considered good news. But the idea that a bunch of heroin addicts, who also happened to be convicted felons, were moving onto the block—well, this quiet little corner of Staten Island went berserk.

The people picketed. They rallied. They petitioned the politicians. They formed an association. They wrote angry letters all over town. They yelled nasty things at the people coming in and out of the house. They seemed genuinely frightened, and their language was harsh.

Daytop Lodge was "a scourge" and "a menace," to use two of the more popular terms of the day. It was a "diabolical invasion," warned one letter-writer in the *Staten Island Advance*. "A hazard to the community," agreed Staten Island District Attorney John M. Braisted, who was campaigning for a third term that fall. Another neighbor was so upset she put up a sign on her front lawn. "I will never accept Daytop," the sign said.

In the November election for city council and district attorney, two acrimonious races, Daytop was the only issue about which all the candidates seemed to agree: This drug-treatment center had to go. Soon, the neighbors had organized themselves in a group called the Butler Manor Vigilance Committee, vowing to eject the "dope pushers" from their "open-door prison."

No one in the neighborhood had yet been attacked, admitted one of the committee's leaders, Heyward White. But, he added: "It must happen, and it will happen. There will be a breakout, and someone in our community will be hurt."

A breakout? This kind of talk produced titters inside the Lodge. The front door, after all, was never locked, day or night. All this commotion—and the headlines that were appearing nearly every day in the *Staten Island Advance*—created a certain excitement inside the Lodge. "We had the clear impression that we were in the vanguard of something, although we didn't quite know what," recalled Bobby Boriello, one of the early crew.

But the uproar caught Shelly and Bassin entirely by surprise. "It never occurred to me that there would be any consequences," Shelly said. "I just wasn't concerned about the people up the street. But this turned out to be an extraordinary case of not-in-my-backyard."

"This was something new, where a community organizes against a treatment facility," Bassin explained. "Now, it happens every ten or fifteen days, whenever any program moves in. But we really weren't prepared for the reaction."

The neighbors suggested an alternate location for Daytop: a small island in the middle of New York Harbor near the Statue of Liberty. "It hadn't been inhabited except by rats for god-knows-how-long," Shelly recalled.

As the months rolled on, the intensity of the neighborhood opposition only grew. Area merchants, who were already doing business with the new program, got jittery. The man at the clothing store in Tottenville had been eager to fill Daytop's first order of tee shirts and khaki pants. But he said no to the second call. "I'd like to do it," he said. "I need the business, and I've got nothing against these people. But I have years of goodwill to protect." The local dairy even cut off Daytop's milk deliveries—agreeing only later to send someone out in an unmarked car.

By May, the neighbors had hired a lawyer. Legal papers were drawn up, demanding that Daytop be closed.

The neighbors advanced two legal theories: that the Brooklyn Probation Department had no legal right to accept federal grant money and that the old Butler mansion was not properly zoned for the treatment of a "contagious disease"—that is, drug addiction.

"My community, formerly serene and peaceful and ideal for family living, is now the scene of sightseers, curiosity seekers, stormy protest marches, uncertainty, panic, hysteria and grave concern among the residents," Butler Boulevard resident James Carmody, one of the plaintiffs, told the Richmond County Supreme Court. Carmody said the Lodge threatened the value of his home and the safety of his children. He did not "want them to become the victim or statistic of some probationer's grave malfeasance."

Shelly went on the offensive. "Thoughtful citizens must be sick at heart to witness the continued hounding of our defenseless young men at Daytop Lodge," Shelly said in his answer to the lawsuit. "These twenty-five probationers, all heavily addicted to heroin before coming to Daytop Lodge, are now off narcotic drugs for the first time in years and well on the road to recovery."

Despite such talk, the Daytop-Must-Go rallies grew larger as the summer wore on. Five hundred people—screaming, some of them throwing rocks at the house and pelting Daytop cars with eggs—turned out for a particularly raucous rally on June 16. An anti-Daytop motorcade wound its way around Staten Island on June 26, and a gigantic rally was held at Tottenville High School on July 20.

This anti-Daytop hostility would continue for years on Staten Island. Similar outrage has erupted just about every time a drug-treatment facility has opened anywhere. But most of those campaigns lose steam eventually, and that's what happened on Staten Island in 1963. The legal challenges were ultimately tossed out of court. The energy of the protesters began to fade. Over time, some of the neighbors ventured into the Lodge for the Saturday-night open houses. Many of them even left impressed.

Indeed, it wasn't the threats from the neighborhood that just about derailed Daytop before it ever got rolling. The real problem is what was going on inside.

Daytop Lodge never was the menace its Staten Island neighbors imagined. None of them was ever attacked or robbed by a Daytop resident. Their children didn't become drug addicts any more quickly than anyone else's children did. Houses in the neighborhood still fetched good prices when they were put up for sale.

So what was the problem?

All the basic ingredients seemed to be in place. The federal money was appropriated. The house was filled with residents. The Synanon-inspired program seemed to be in place. But still, something very big was wrong.

The residents, all street-smart heroin addicts, quickly figured out how to twist the Daytop structure to their own convenience. Before long, they were sneaking alcohol and drugs into the house. They were making compacts not to report each other's transgressions. And when the occasional drug tests were scheduled, the residents were trading urine samples like baseball cards.

"The probation department and the staff people they hired, their hearts were all in the right place," said Bobby Boriello. "They did the best they could. But they underestimated the manipulative power of a houseful of New York junkies."

The residents kept up appearances, most of the time. They showed up as they were supposed to for the group seminars and the encounter sessions. All of them could talk earnestly about the importance of living drug free. Then, when the Colcords went off to sleep at night, big, fat joints would be brought down from the bedrooms. Or someone would slip into Tottenville and come back with bottles of Thunderbird.

From the time he arrived, Boriello remembered, "I knew everybody was getting high." One evening, he cornered one of the older residents. "I said, 'I want to be in on some of this.' And he said, 'Just be cool. You're brand new. Stick around a little while.'" He didn't have to wait long.

"We sort of had an agreement," Charlie Devlin remembered. "We saw this was a good thing, and in our way we wanted to do what was right. We said there will be no heroin use, no goofball use. But it was okay to smoke a little bit of pot. To us smoking pot was like drinking, like having a bottle of beer. And it was okay to drink. And there was the contract that nobody would say anything about each other."

"The residents had basically the same values as the penitentiary,"

Boriello said. "The black people looked out for the black people. The white people looked out for the white people. The attitude was, well, we'll play their game for a little while, and we'll all get out of doing time."

One of the things that made this especially easy was the man Shelly and Bassin had hired to run Daytop Lodge. The man they hired, Dean Colcord, looked a little like Chuck Dederich, the revered founder of Synanon, and he too was an alcoholic from AA. But Colcord had none of Dederich's charisma and none of Dederich's shrewdness. He turned out to be no match for the people he was hired to save.

"Dean was a very sweet, kind man," said Alex Bassin, who hired him. "But he would call me up at one or two o'clock in the morning, about how the kids were torturing him and how they were torturing his wife Linda. They would delight at making fun of her. They would call her crazy. It's unbelievable what these kids were capable of."

As assistant director of the Lodge, Colcord had hired a physician from Massachusetts who had lost his license because of his drinking and drug use. The fallen physician still liked to be called "Doc." He was a compassionate man, and many of the residents preferred him to the stiffer Dean Colcord. Colcord sensed that. Before long, the two were at each other's throats. And both of them were confiding their unhappiness to Bassin.

He recalled: "I would hold Dean's hand and say, 'Don't give up. Keep on trying.' And I would speak to Doc and say, 'Please don't fight so much. It doesn't look good for you two grown-ups to be fighting.' Dean's wife would be crying to me about how all the kids were tormenting her. And the kids were having a great time."

Charlie Devlin was often the "night man" in those days, responsible for staying up late and keeping an eye on things. Doc also kept late hours. "He would talk with me for hours, ramble on and on and on," Devlin said. "Well, I knew right away this old cuss was getting high."

Devlin didn't turn Doc in. But one day when Doc was out of the house, Devlin snuck into the older man's bedroom and found a stash of pills. "There must have been at least a thousand of these pills," Devlin said. "It turns out they were sodium pentothal. I grabbed a handful, put them in my pocket. Then, I did the obvious. I started taking them, too."

Doc didn't last much longer. He made a public, drunken scene one day at Rockefeller Center and was told to find another job.

Things were sufficiently out of hand by then that Shelly and Bassin were getting nervous. "The residents were dominating the house," Bassin said. "They were very smart. Cunning, sharp, con men. They had all lived out on the street, supporting expensive drug habits. Most of them had done time in jail. It became obvious that Dean didn't have control over the place. He finally said, 'I can't take it.' We started looking for somebody else."

Shelly interviewed the candidates. But it didn't prove easy. No one really knew much then about using group therapy to treat addicts. Chuck Dederich, the man who had invented most of it, was refusing to help. To make matters even worse, the job didn't pay that well. The result: over the next nine months, Daytop Lodge was directed by seven different people. Not one of them got it right.

One was a social worker who was so terrorized by the residents he snuck out a window in the middle of the night—and did not return. Another had been the commandant of a military academy on the north shore of Long Island. The school had gone out of business. He was well spoken and had an impressive military bearing. "He turned out to be a dud," Shelly remembered. "The kids back at his school might have been a little maladjusted, but this was something else entirely."

Then there was the twenty-five-year-old doctoral candidate in sociology, who came with glowing recommendations. But he and Shelly got into a bitter fight when the young man took one of the newer residents out for $1,200 worth of dental work—without getting clearance first. "To us, that was a stupendous sum of money,"

Shelly said. "When we heard that, we hit the ceiling." The graduate student was gone the next week.

Another one was a heavyset young man who kept hypodermic needles in his room. About a month after he was bounced, he was found dead of a heroin overdose. And there was the director with the severe credit problems. His car was repossessed from the Daytop driveway. He was gone soon after that.

As this parade of failed directors was moving in and out of the house, the residents were consolidating their control. After a while, they were even interviewing the candidates for director. "We knew they needed us because they always reminded us how important we were, how the success of the program relied on us," Devlin said. "Before you knew it, we pretty much were running the place and making the decisions about what went on."

MAKING IT WORK **6**

The greatest thing in this world is not so much where we are, but in what direction we are moving.

—Oliver Wendell Holmes

At the same time Shelly and Bassin were flailing around with their experiment on Staten Island, Dan Casriel and I were doing some flailing of our own.

Most of our energy was still devoted to Synanon, the California program that had invented this remarkable new approach to treating drug addicts. We were among Synanon's biggest boosters. As we had for several years, we were raising money for the group and helping recruit addicts from the New York area—then as now the number-one drug-impact zone in America.

Eventually both Casriel and I lost faith in Synanon. But there is no denying the group's amazing accomplishments or how it revolutionized the treatment of hard-core drug addicts.

Synanon's founder, Chuck Dederich, had succeeded where everyone else had failed. He recognized that, with the proper support, addicts could truly find the motivation to cure themselves. The proof of Dederich's success lay in Synanon's graduates, hundreds of people who went from severe drug addiction to truly productive lives. By the early 1960s, Dederich had gotten a tremendous amount of acclaim, prodded along by his remarkable gift for self-promotion.

Gradually, however, disturbing signs began to appear.

Dederich began speaking of himself in the third person, as the all-powerful force. He began describing Synanon as the one pure and moral place in the universe. The rest of the world, he said, was irredeemably corrupt. Even more frightening, he began redefining Synanon as a lifelong commitment, a cradle-to-grave community that residents should never expect to leave.

His rhetoric about the evils of the outside world grew darker and more strident. At the same time, he was willing to tolerate— even to encourage—greater and greater levels of violence and repression inside the group. The Synanon resident or staff member who would question even the smallest edict from "the old man," as he liked to call himself, risked being labeled a vicious enemy of the community.

This crazy talk was in full force by early 1964.

By then, Casriel and I had already had several spirited arguments between ourselves about Synanon. He reminded me, correctly, of Dederich's genius and of his great accomplishments. I expressed growing doubts. And as the year wore on, both of us became deeply concerned.

Several times, I tried expressing these misgivings to Dederich and his top lieutenants out in California.

At first, they acted interested in my critiques and gave earnest, reasonable-sounding explanations for whatever particular issue I had raised. But as I pressed on with my questions, the Californians grew downright defensive. "You're selling us out," I was told more than once. "You're giving up on the Synanon ideal."

The truth is that, if anything, I was too slow to back away. Dederich had a tremendous reservoir of goodwill among his East Coast supporters, and he was not eager to lose it. We did, after all, provide him with money and fresh recruits—two things for which Dederich had an unquenchable thirst.

The growing tensions between us finally blew up in September of 1964.

To quiet our complaints, Dederich had agreed to come to New York and meet with us. A meeting was set up at Casriel's apartment on Seventy-second Street in Manhattan. Dederich was coming, along with his top aide, Reid Kimball. Casriel and I and several other long-time Synanon supporters were also going to be there.

But Dederich didn't show. He sent Kimball alone. That wasn't what we had wanted. But this, apparently, was all we were going to get.

Casriel and I laid out for him five specific objections to what had been going on at Synanon—things that, in our view, were simply intolerable.

First, we told Kimball, Synanon could not be "for life." The idea, we always believed, was for addicts to spend a limited time in treatment and then return to the real world, better able to cope.

Second, we explained, we believed that Synanon's methods ought to be scrutinized by outside researchers. We were confident that Dederich was truly on to something. So why not let the world confirm and understand it? What was he trying to hide?

Third, we wanted to know, shouldn't Synanon at least consider the insights of professionals? What was Synanon scared of? If the problems of drug abuse in America are ever going to be solved, we argued to Kimball, the response had to be a coordinated one. Doesn't the "whole person" need to be healed? So why not form a team of helping professionals and let everyone play a role?

Our fourth objection had to do with Synanon's increasingly harsh disciplinary techniques. This had gotten way out of hand. We doubted the therapeutic value, for instance, of dunking people into cesspools, one Dederich favorite. Humiliation seemed to be the only point.

Finally, we told Kimball, if Synanon was going to thrive, it would have to come to New York. New York, we reminded him, had by far the biggest drug problem in America. Somehow or other, Synanon had to make its impact felt in the main arena. And succeeding in New York meant establishing a responsible, businesslike posture to administer public funds.

Kimball listened, obviously distracted, as Casriel and then I spoke.

When we were done, he proceeded to tell us "no way" on all five counts.

And he let loose a barrage of invective—"You are despicable

sell-outs!" "You are too stupid to understand what Chuck is trying to do!" "We don't need your infantile complaints!"—that chased me right out of the room.

Casriel had a little more patience. But before too much longer, he showed Kimball to the door.

Synanon, Casriel and I agreed when we spoke the next morning, was hopeless. The writing was already on the wall: Synanon would devour itself. If we intended to keep working on the problems of drug abuse—and we knew that we did—we had to start doing things for ourselves.

That's when we decided to go see Mayor Robert Wagner.

Wagner had always been supportive of our efforts in the Bronx, showing up at fund raisers and making his drug experts available to us.

When I called city hall for an appointment, the mayor got right on the phone and urged Casriel and me to come down for a chat.

We gave Wagner a quick replay of our disenchantment with Synanon. We spared him the usual sales pitch on the need for drug treatment. He already knew all that.

"So what do you want to do?" he asked, after listening for a few minutes to our litany of Synanon complaints.

That was our opening, and we grabbed it.

Casriel and I laid out for him just the kind of treatment program we wanted to establish. It would take advantage of some of Synanon's insights but would include iron-clad protections against the sort of excesses that Dederich had wrought.

We were talking about a long-term, residential treatment program, but with enough flexibility to deal with the ever-changing face of drug abuse. The program would need enough independence to operate creatively. But we were not nearly as suspicious of government help as Dederich was. If this complex problem of drug abuse is ever going to be licked, we reminded the mayor, government would have to be part of the plan.

Wagner looked intrigued. But he toyed with us a little first. "Look at this," he said.

He was pointing to a bookshelf behind his desk.

"Thirty-four years," he continued. "Thirty-four years of reports on what to do about drugs in New York. People look at all those reports, and they think the problem must be hopeless. Maybe they're right. And maybe I'm being a fool, but I don't believe that. Go ahead. You have my support. I'll try and help you get some money. See what you can do."

Then, he was quiet for a second. "Remember those thirty-four years of reports," he said. "It's a tough fight. But I believe in you. I think you can make it work."

We spent another hour with the mayor, talking specifics.

Casriel was quite familiar with the probation department's efforts on Staten Island. He was still stopping by the Lodge for his weekly visits, and he knew just how frustrated Shelly and Bassin were. Casriel was the one who brought up the idea of somehow linking our interest to theirs.

Wagner didn't need to be told of the program's shortcomings. And he said that the probation department was looking for a way to bow out gracefully that might still salvage something from all their work. We were eager to provide a vehicle for that.

Within twenty-four hours, we had established Daytop Village, the first of the second-generation therapeutic communities to get off the ground.

Now, instead of trying to convince Chuck Dederich to open his mind, all of our caveats were built in from the start.

This was our show, and we proceeded to pick up the pieces from the probation department and try to construct a program that could be sustained.

The focus would now be broader than just probationers. Addicts, we knew, came from all sorts of backgrounds. We didn't want to limit the focus of our program. For that reason, we knew women should be welcomed as residents, as well.

We had no problem with the Daytop name, although we did need to fiddle a bit with the words behind the acronym. It was no longer accurate to describe the program as Drug Addicts Treated on Probation. So we fudged the words and came up with this: Drug Addicts Yielding to Persuasion.

And we were hoping that Daytop might one day become a truly wide-ranging program. We didn't know how wide, but we knew we wanted something bigger than the one house on Staten Island. So "Lodge" wouldn't do so well either, we thought. "Village," we decided, was really more of what we had in mind.

Daytop Village.

Casriel became the supervising psychiatrist. I set up the board of directors. But we still needed someone to run the place.

Almost simultaneously, Casriel and I remembered our old friend David Deitch, the charismatic ex-addict from Chicago we had met that day in Westport. Back then, he had been one of Dederich's most trusted lieutenants. But we had heard that, more recently, he too had grown disenchanted with "the old man" and with Synanon's rapid slide into craziness. He had been called back to California a couple of times and reamed out by Dederich. By the time Casriel called him, he was back in Connecticut, living in a rented room in someone's attic, more or less estranged from Synanon.

He thought about our offer for about five minutes, then readily agreed to become the first director of Daytop Village.

We were off and running.

Deitch was a wiry young man, with thick glasses and a gaze as intense as a cobra's. His attire was always casual, and he spoke with an accent that was right off the street corners of Chicago. But he had a way about him—one-on-one, or with a large group—that was absolutely spellbinding. The man oozed real.

He had made a terrific impression on Casriel and me that day up in Westport and at our various meetings after that. But neither of us was truly prepared for his performance the day he was introduced to the twenty-five residents at the Staten Island Daytop house.

Before actually taking over, Deitch had slipped in and out of the house a few times, discreetly watching the residents and engaging in casual-seeming small-talk. As a former heroin addict with all those years at Synanon, it did not take him long to get a fix on the program's woes. He could tell right away that, whatever the staff might think, it was the resident addicts who were really in charge.

But he didn't say a word about any of this until the whole group was called together one morning, and he was introduced as their new director—the ninth or tenth of the year.

A few rumors had circulated through the group about Deitch coming from Synanon, a name all the residents knew. But I don't think anyone was expecting an awful lot.

That was a big mistake.

Deitch began speaking in a flat and quiet tone.

He introduced himself. He told a little about his own background—his childhood in suburban Skokie, Illinois, his long heroin addiction, his recovery at Synanon, his rise in the organization and his time as director of the Westport house.

He was getting started slowly and gauging the temperature of the room. He could sense the familiar smugness of the addict audience, men who had perfected their own personal cons and were sure those cons would work forever.

Then, he got down to business.

"You people are a bunch of frauds," he said.

Several people in the room looked a little startled by this sudden shift in tone.

"I know what's been going on here," he continued. "You know what's been going on. It's disgraceful, and it will change. It will change quickly, and it will change dramatically. You can be part of that change. Or you can get out."

Daytop residents were not used to being spoken to like that. The past directors had all been far more circumspect—too insecure or too intimidated to confront the residents head on.

There were a few more perplexed looks in the room and even a few muffled giggles. But Deitch didn't let any of this shake his concentration.

"The first thing you've got to do is admit what's been going on here," he said. Still, he had never said exactly what he was referring to. But you could tell by the looks around the room that his listeners knew—and they knew that he knew.

"Then, you've got to pay," he said. "We are going to begin that process right now. If it takes five hours, or ten hours, we are going to give it up."

It took about twelve.

"This is not a joke," Deitch said solemnly. "This is not about going through the motions. This is about saving your lives."

Looking back on it now, much of Deitch's rhetoric that day was not so different from the things that the previous directors had tried to say. Somehow, though, out of his mouth, it seemed to connect.

"Give it up," he said finally. "Give it up. Give it up."

And they did.

First, one resident went upstairs and came back with an empty wine bottle. Deitch ordered the young man to put the bottle in the middle of the floor.

Someone else went upstairs and got a small baggie of marijuana and some cigarette papers.

"Let me see the stash," Deitch demanded.

He inspected the pot and the papers, and then threw them disgustedly onto the living-room floor, right next to the wine bottle.

It went on like this for hours.

In the end, the living-room floor was littered with a big pile of contraband, symbols of all the ways the house had been out of control. More importantly, that pile was a symbol of how things would be run from then on.

Not everyone responded well to the new order.

One resident got up quietly and walked out the back door.

"Fuck this," another resident said disgustedly, and he too stormed out.

But everyone else stayed put.

The day David Deitch arrived was the day Daytop really began to work. He brought to us the one thing that we had most sorely needed—a director who could not be conned. And over the months that followed, Deitch, with help of several others, began to create a Daytop that in most ways resembles the place we know today.

Some of it was borrowed from Synanon and Alcoholics Anonymous and other places that we came to know. Some of it was dreamed up by those of us who were there at the time—including both residents and staff. And some of it just sort of grew, organically, over the years. We kept the things that worked. We discarded the things that didn't. None of it happened instantly. But, before long, we had a program that made a certain amount of internal sense.

Over the decades that followed, Daytop Village experienced many, many challenges. Some were the results of our shortcomings. Some were the results of our truly unexpected success.

But in the end, not only did we survive, we thrived.

These years have been a time of almost constant expansion—and many lessons learned.

We knew from the beginning that the old Butler mansion was not going to accommodate us. So, right away, we went looking for larger quarters. What we found was a rambling beachfront building on Prince's Bay in Staten Island, about a mile from the old Butler house.

By the mid-1960s, it became clear that Daytop would have to grow beyond one house on Staten Island, no matter how commodious that house might be. This was the beginning of America's drug explosion, the era of Woodstock and Hendrix and Joplin. The upward mobility of drug use was becoming increasingly hard to ignore.

Daytop had gotten some press in the New York area. Local judges and probation officers were calling constantly. Far too often, we simply had no room at the inn.

So we began looking to expand.

Logistically, Staten Island had some drawbacks as a location for a residential drug-treatment program. Not for the reasons that our angry neighbors were constantly citing—that our residents were going to corrupt the island's children, spoil its beaches and depress its property values. We never did any of those things, even in the first, rocky year of Daytop Lodge.

But we had come to recognize several advantages to operating in a more rural setting, which Staten Island decidedly was not. Distance from the drug-ridden streets was one advantage. A bigger one was that the country offered us more room to grow.

Our search led us first to the Catskill Mountains, an aging resort community north of New York City that, to put it kindly, had seen better days. The landscape was beautiful. The proximity to the city was a plus. And the reasonable real-estate prices brought the region into our reach.

We bought—were given, really—the old Paul's Hotel in Swan Lake, which had gone out of business a few years before. The place was not in great shape. Built as a summer retreat for city dwellers, it didn't even have a heating system. But the property was spacious. And the price was right.

We had all the expected opposition—from the neighboring land-owners, the region's hotel association and the local press. But with hard work and important assists from a few good-hearted citizens who understood what we were trying to do, Daytop's first upstate house opened June 14, 1966, and the residents began moving in.

In the years that followed, I am proud to say, Daytop has continued to expand its facilities and its programs, responding creatively to the ever-changing face of drug abuse. Today, we have eight Daytop houses, and we are making plans for more.

We came in the late 1960s to recognize that, despite our strong commitment to the idea of residential treatment, it wasn't right for every user. So Daytop opened a network of storefront Outreach Centers—then called SPAN (Special Project Against Neglect) Centers—through the New York City area.

The Outreach Centers, as they came to be called, had a dual purpose: They allowed someone literally to walk off the street and get help with a drug problem. And since the centers were staffed by senior Daytop residents, they provided a valuable bridge between life inside and out.

Having an urban street presence was especially important as our residential centers were being established out in the countryside. It gave city dwellers a chance to actually see some of the work that Daytop did.

Originally, the idea was funded by the U.S. Office of Economic Opportunity in Washington. But the walk-in centers proved so valuable that we were able to raise other funding when the federal money ran out. Ultimately, we expanded the idea throughout the metropolitan area.

We now have Outreach Centers in all five boroughs of New York City—Manhattan, Brooklyn, the Bronx, Queens and Staten Island—and in Nassau, Suffolk, Westchester, and Rockland counties to serve the suburbs.

And that's not all. This same sense of broadened mission has led to our expanding the notion of drug treatment well beyond its traditional bounds.

Early on, we saw a need to include the addict's family in the treatment. The Daytop Family Association was formed in 1966 and has thousands of members today—contributing immeasurably to their loved ones' recovery and healing themselves in the bargain.

At each step of our history, we have learned as much from our failures as from our successes. It took us a full decade, for instance, to recognize that women were not getting their fair share from Daytop treatment. Daytop had emerged from the macho world of urban heroin addiction and, in the early years, still had a largely male population. Daytop women too often found themselves walking an uncomfortable line: They were being accused of flaunting their sexuality, or they had to so repress their female side that their own true needs weren't being met.

The women complained about this, and we were too slow to listen to their frustration and pain. Finally though, they succeeded in opening our minds. We came to understand how an equal role for women is a vital part of our community treatment. On the outside, all our residents will have to learn to live harmoniously with both women and men. There is no reason not to begin teaching those lessons in treatment.

The result of this belated understanding is a distinct and integral Women's Treatment Program, piloted by Vice President Tish Zingale, along with staff mentor Maxine Thomas. Since 1975, women at Daytop have been thoroughly integrated into the regular treatment program. And we have been making added efforts to deal with their particular concerns through special groups and retreats. I think most residents today would agree that Daytop is finally a "woman-friendly" place.

We've always felt that Daytop residents should give back to the community they live in. That's the idea behind the Daytop C.A.R.E.S. program. Executive Vice President Brian Madden chartered this caring mission for us. It's been going strong since 1979, providing meals and other services to elderly shut-ins. The old people benefit. So do we. The relationships that grow up teach wonderful lessons about helping others and truly loving our neighbors in a Christ-like way.

Dozens of other such programs have grown up inside Daytop over the years. The Daytop Mini-versity allows our residents to earn college credits during treatment, a creation of Vice President Yasser Hijasi and Research Director Vincent Biase. The Art-Feeling Workshop, patterned on the theories of Jackson Pollock and directed by Susan Rizzo, has opened new and creative frontiers for personal expression through color, tint, shape, and form. Miracles have un-folded there.

There is now a special program for residents who are HIV pos-itive, dealing with an especially hard-to-reach population. Daytop's chief of medicine, Dr. Azimer Ehr, has fashioned a monumental breakthrough. Another Daytop program is designed for pregnant addicts. It has shown amazing success in preventing one of the most heart-rending occurrences imaginable—the birth of a drug-ad-dicted infant. Pregnant addicts are actually giving up drugs and delivering healthy babies. This is the brainchild of Delia Campbell.

You'd need a scorecard to keep track of all the facilities we've rented, bought and sold over the years to keep up with this ever-growing demand: a separate Re-entry Center opened on Fourteenth Street in 1969, the Millbrook House for adolescents in 1971, the Parksville House for adults in 1972, a headquarters building at 54 West Fortieth Street in Manhattan the same year, the new Entry and Re-entry Center in Far Rockaway, Queens, in 1984; the Rhinebeck Campus in 1979, Daytop's largest Upstate facility, encompassing four distinct facilities, the Springwood Campus, Fox Run Campus, Meadow Run Campus, and Brightside Lodge.

The list goes on and on.

In 1987, through the generosity of Bill Wackenfeld and the Hay-den Foundation, we opened the Promethean Center in Milford, Pennsylvania, a central site for staff training and other educational programs. In 1988, we started our first center in California, with Daytops in Redwood City, East Palo Alto and Belmont. The following year, we managed to open an Outreach Center in Dallas, followed by twin residential centers outside Houston and Dallas.

And no one has even suggested stopping there. The need is simply too great.

FORCING THE CHANGE **7**

We, too, may have the greatest resistance to admitting that alcohol, and all the term implies, is only a metaphor for innumerable, interrelated dependencies. Without being conscious of it, we subject ourselves to the dependencies on a daily basis to help us avoid pain, difficulty and discomfort generated by our pursuit of pleasure. Alcohol becomes quite simply a synonym for self-deception, self-betrayal, living a lie. All the while, the alcoholic or addict is only the smoke that tells us that there is a fire somewhere. We try to make the smoke go away and content ourselves with that. But the alcoholic and addict shows us again and again in penetrating, disturbing and in unbearable ways, that something smells—somewhere—something in us.

—Walther H. Lechler, M.D., 1991 Symposium,
Promethean Institute, Milford, Pennsylvania

Addicts don't simply wake up one morning and decide on their own to stop using drugs. It just doesn't happen like that. Waiting around for an addict's epiphany is nothing but a waste of time. The day will never come. The addict will die first. Or he'll destroy himself. Surely, he'll destroy the people who love him. In the meantime, the things he'll do to get the drugs he craves will grow more and more degrading, more and more extreme.

Human beings suffer from a huge array of diseases: cancer, heart failure, Parkinson's, muscular dystrophy—the list goes on and on. Yet drug and alcohol addictions are just about the only ailments that the patients do not suffer from. They enjoy their afflictions. The pain comes from not having the substances they love. And it is this love of the affliction, more than anything else, that makes curing addicts so frustratingly difficult.

Over the years, thousands of parents have come up to me—tears in their eyes, their families torn apart by the awful cruelties that an addicted son or daughter can inflict. "We're waiting for the kid to grow out of it," the parents will say. Or, "Father, we're hoping and praying she'll see what the drugs are doing to her."

Not a chance.

Invariably, these parents are good, well-meaning people, who want only the best for their kids. But a drug addict? Just stop? Highly unlikely. These parents don't know what they are up against. Their stoic optimism is touching. But it completely fails to grasp the drug addict's mind.

Given a choice, most addicts will continue using drugs forever. And the physical pangs they periodically experience pale against the exhilaration of getting high. The simple truth is that addicts love their drugs. They love their drugs more than they love their families, more than they love their own lives. Drugs are an addict's best friend, an addict's lover, a magic wand that an addict has to take all the bad things in life and make them disappear—if only for a little while.

"Ever since I first started using, people were warning me about all the things drugs could do to me," said Marvin, a lanky, former high-school point guard who shot heroin for twenty-two of his thirty-eight years. "They were right. I know that now. But every time they'd be talking, I'd be thinking: 'To me? It's what they're doing *for* me, all these warm feelings the drugs have inside them.'

"Drugs were the only thing I cared about. And for all those years, I actually believed the drugs cared about me."

You can't expect someone to walk blithely away from that. And it's not enough to remind the addict about all the damage the drugs have caused—the ruined health, the desperate finances, the fractured friendships and families, the loss of schooling and jobs, the bouts with the police and the courts. At times, the addict may feel bad about these things, but never bad enough to give up the drugs for good. The grip is just too strong.

Addicts are always making promises to the people who care about them, wonderful-sounding promises. "I'll do something about my problem," the addict will say. "I'll make that call tomorrow."

Nearly every drug addict I've ever known has made that promise at one time or another, often after being confronted by a worried relative or friend. Some of them even believe themselves. Then, tomorrow comes. And a different kind of drug problem has pushed to the front of the addict's mind: how to score another bag of heroin, another vial of crack, another gram of cocaine.

Terrific intentions. Postponed results. Serious drug addicts can keep that pattern going for years. They can see themselves spiraling downward. They genuinely intend to change their lives. But a drug that has turned into an addiction, they find, is terribly hard to drop.

"In the last years I was using," Marvin recalled, "I just about got into a program a whole lot of times. Something always came up to stop me. What came up was usually another bag of dope."

Think of addiction like a toothache. For most of us, a toothache is a manageable problem—excruciating perhaps, but manageable. The tooth hurts, so we telephone the dentist's office and set up an appointment. We show up for the appointment. The dentist does whatever it is he does. Chances are, the toothache goes away.

This sequence is relatively simple, something most of us are able to follow in most parts of our lives. But some people get sidetracked. For them, the tooth aches. They recognize the pain for what it is. They understand that the dentist is the person who can help ease it. They might even telephone for an appointment. Then, briefly, the tooth stops aching. The dentist is forgotten. The urgency is gone. Yet just beneath the gum line, the abscess lingers, growing more infected by the minute, sure to erupt again in agony in a matter of hours or days.

That's what happens when most addicts confront their drug use.

They recognize the problem that drugs have become—even when they keep that recognition to themselves. "I'm going to get myself into treatment," they'll promise a relative or a friend at some moment when drugs have fallen into short supply. "I'll make the call tomorrow." But by the time the appointment comes around, they've found the drugs they were aching for. All memory of that promise has disappeared.

What happened in Marvin's case is that he got arrested again, for what must have been the twenty-fifth time. He had been picked up many times before on drug-possession charges and even had a couple of arrests for small drug sales. His rap sheet also included a few burglaries, some larcenies, and one minor assault.

But this time, guns had come out in a drug deal, and an under-cover cop was in the room. Marvin didn't have one of the weapons, but he was dragged down to the precinct with everyone else.

"If I really had a choice, I don't think I ever would have come to Daytop," he said. "The judge laid it on the line for me. I was going Upstate 'one way or the other,' he told me. Did I want to do my time in prison? Or did I want to try to get a grip on my problem and go in to Daytop instead?

"I figured this was probably my last chance, and I sure didn't want to go back to jail. I had a problem with probation, so the sentence would have been real long. I just told myself, 'Do it now, or you're gonna be dead.' "

It is important to remember why drug addicts finally do something about their problem. They do it because of external pressure to do it *today*. Almost always, some great crisis has to occur before tomorrow is turned into today.

Maybe the crisis is an arrest, as in Marvin's case. Thirty-eight percent of our residents end up at Daytop that way. They get arrested for some crime or another, and the judge offers a choice: Go to Daytop or go to jail.

In some cases, the crisis was created by a spouse or a parent, whose patience was finally gone. "Get out of the house this instant," they said. Or, "I'm leaving you if you don't get help." In other instances, the boss at work was the one to deliver the ultimatum: "The drugs are destroying your performance. Get help now, or you're out of here for good."

Almost always, it's something like that. Remember, addicts don't just renounce their addictions. Some outside force has to be so compelling that it overcomes the powerful draw of drugs—and pushes the addict into action *today*.

Over the past thirty years, more than 75,000 adults and teenagers have come to Daytop for help with a drug problem. I don't believe more than a few of them ever walked entirely voluntarily through the door. Somehow or other, every one felt pushed.

This isn't to say we drag people kicking and screaming into Daytop. For several reasons, that's a bad idea—the federal laws against kidnaping being only the most obvious. It also doesn't work. Recovering from drug addiction is a rough and demanding process, which in the end cannot be forced on someone else. We work hard to show our residents why they should want to escape from the life of the needle or the pipe. We work even harder to convince them that they are capable of living without drugs. But in the end, Daytop does not stop drug addiction. With Daytop's help, drug addicts learn to help themselves.

What this means is that a balance must be achieved between the coerced and the free. Addicts seek treatment only when they've decided it's the only choice they have. And this will never happen until their other choices start looking pretty bleak.

"To be honest with you, if it hadn't been for the HIV, I don't think I ever would have come," said Larry, a forty-three-year-old heroin addict who had been shooting drugs on the Lower East Side of Manhattan since he dropped out of high school at sixteen.

His case is an extreme one. But to a greater or lesser extent, the theme fits just about everyone who ever comes to Daytop.

"I was living in an abandoned building," he said. "I didn't really mind that. I had to spend all my time hustling for money. I didn't mind that too much either. Shooting drugs, I've seen all kinds of people overdose and die and a lot of terrible things. I figured, 'Well, it hadn't happened to me yet, so I'm all right.' I have been in jail so many times I don't even remember."

Larry put up with it all.

Finally, he got the AIDS virus—from sharing dirty needles, he thinks. It wasn't until the doctor told him the diagnosis that he gave any serious thought to trying to get off the drugs.

"I guess I had to hit bottom," he said. "Sometimes that's necessary, you know, before you can start going up."

That's always been one of the basic tenets at Alcoholics Anonymous, and it was a lesson I learned over the years from the many AA people I came to know.

One of them was the Broadway theater giant Frank Fay, whom I got to know when I was a young priest at St. Patrick's Cathedral. Another was the early radio and TV personality Walter O'Keefe. Both men had been problem drinkers and had achieved sobriety with AA.

Both of them used to say that your pride must go before you can climb the steep hill toward recovery. The AA saying went something like this: "Your chin in the gutter, resting on concrete, is the ultimate wipe-out of pride—no one below to look down on or lord over."

Hitting bottom is the key to humility and the launching pad toward recovery. It's as true today as it was back then and as true for drug addicts as it is for alcoholics.

Typically, the process starts with a telephone call.

Daytop's Pre-screen Unit is located on the third floor of our center in Far Rockaway, Queens. When someone with a drug problem phones out of the blue, Pre-screen is where the call is sent.

Every week, we get hundreds of such calls. Steve Conforte, a former cocaine addict with long curly hair and a disarmingly direct manner, is usually the person who picks up the phone.

"Hello, Daytop, may I help you? Would you hold, please?"

"Hello, Daytop. One moment, please."

"Hello, Daytop, may I help you? I have to put you on hold for a second. Be right back to you."

"Hi, I'm sorry to keep you waiting."

The beige, six-line phone on Steve's desk buzzes like that all through the day and night. Sometimes, it's a relative calling. "My son," the voice will say, quaking so much that the words are hard to make out. Sometimes, it's a social worker, a probation officer, a jail counselor, a defense lawyer or someone else from the so-called helping professions. Those calls usually start out on a more clinical note. "I have a client in need of services," the voice will say. Or, "How long is Daytop's waiting list right now?"

Most often, though, the voice on the other end of the line belongs to someone in serious trouble, someone whose life has been wrecked by drugs. The plea gets phrased a thousand different ways. The tone might be nervous, or angry, or desperate, or icily cold. But one way or another, the message comes across: "I need help."

Steve's job is to figure out in a few seconds whether the caller is a potential candidate for Daytop. If so, Steve will ask for some basic information—name, age, address, what kinds of drugs the person is using, that sort of thing. Then, he will invite the caller in for a "pre-screen interview." In general, if the person is at least fifteen years old, has a problem with drug use and expresses some interest in getting help, Steve will give the person an appointment.

"I say, 'Let them show us how serious they are,' " Steve explains.

Because of the incredible volume of calls we get, the interview date might be three or four weeks away. And then, the person just comes for a preliminary screening: brief meetings with counselors from Daytop's admission, legal, medical, and financial offices. Even if the interviews go beautifully and the person is eager to begin treatment, it could easily take another month or two before a bed opens up.

The mathematics here can be exceedingly cruel. There simply isn't enough room at Daytop. We do our absolute best to squeeze people in. We juggle as much as possible. We are constantly trying to expand. And still we never have anywhere near enough room.

Steve Conforte explains this as gently as possible to the people on the telephone. He tells them to try to be patient. And he urges them to start attending night-time groups at one of Daytop's eight Outreach Centers in the New York metropolitan area, while they wait for their "bed dates" to arrive.

The result of all of this is that we lose far too many people in the time it takes to get them through the door. This is one of the most frustrating and depressing facts of life at Daytop. And the problem isn't getting any better. If anything, like the overall drug problem in America, it's only getting worse.

People have done some extraordinary things to get into Daytop.

They beg and plead. They insist and demand. Parents have offered us huge sums of money to get a son or a daughter to the top of the waiting list. Some people have their friends or employers call us. Others ask local clergymen or politicians to lend a hand.

None of this is necessary. Our admissions process is a relatively straightforward affair. We want to be sure that Daytop has something to offer the applicant and that the person is willing to give it a serious try. After that, people get in pretty much on a first-come-first-served basis. Our fees are set on a sliding scale, for those clients who pay at all. So we never reject anyone because of inability to pay.

Still, it is hard not to be touched by the eagerness of some applicants. I remember one boy who had already been interviewed and accepted for treatment. But when the day came for him to appear at the Entry Unit, he didn't have enough money for the subway fare. He had been attending weekly groups at the Daytop Outreach Center in the Bronx. So he had an idea of how much we value honesty, and he didn't want to just sneak onto the train.

He left his parents' home in the North Bronx a little after midnight. That would give him enough time, he figured, to hoof it to the Daytop center in Queens in time for his 9:00 A.M. appointment. In fact, the hike took seven hours, and he told me later that he didn't mind it one bit. "I would have walked to California," he said, "if that's what it took to save my life."

Years ago, before the drug problem had reached its current proportions, the line at Daytop's front door was not nearly so long. But even back then, we always made the applicants work a little to get inside. We had the idea that no one should walk in to Daytop too thoughtlessly. We wanted the newcomers to show us some evidence that they really wanted to join our family.

"Making an investment in your own recovery," we call it. That's always been part of the Daytop philosophy. Today, just getting to the top of the waiting list shows a certain seriousness of purpose. In the old days, we accomplished the same thing with a series of seemingly endless telephone calls. If someone came to me, usually referred by some other clergyman or a teacher or a parent, I would have the young person come in and make a phone call to the Daytop Entry Unit.

From the very first call, the Daytop staff member on the other end of the phone would be filling out an information card. The staff member would tell the person to call back again, usually an hour earlier the following day. In a sense, preliminary treatment had already begun.

After the fifth or sixth day, the hour might be two or three in the morning. If the caller didn't phone at the exact time that was scheduled, the Daytop staffer would refuse to take the call and start the whole process over again.

This might sound like a harsh way to recruit drug addicts into a drug-treatment program. But torture was not the point of the exercise. The idea was to ease the young person into a vertical position, so real treatment could begin. We wanted the addict to begin taking some small steps toward personal responsibility. We wanted that tiny investment for the privilege of coming inside.

Finally, after a series of phone calls, the Daytop staff member would say, "Okay, your appointment is tomorrow morning at eight A.M. Don't come in at five to eight, or five after. Come in right at eight o'clock.

"And by the way, you're off drugs as of now."

This would often be greeted by silence on the other end of the phone. The caller had obviously been taken aback.

"What? I don't know. I'm not sure whether I can do that."

The staff member would answer calmly, "Well, don't bother coming in unless—as of this moment—you've stopped using drugs." Again, we were trying to get the addict vertical, so treatment could begin.

And then the staffer would give a little encouragement to the addict on the other end of the line. "I'm a Daytop graduate. I did it before coming in. It wasn't easy for me, either. But the hard things are best. I wanted to get my life back more than anything. How about you?"

Arrangements would be made for the parents or a friend to bring the caller in, or I would do it myself. We'd drive over to the Entry Unit. We would wait together in the car until a minute before eight. Then, we would walk into the building together at exactly eight o'clock.

The sponsor—whoever it was—would be welcomed at the front desk by the coordinator on duty. The young person would also be greeted and then told, "Sit over there on that chair. That's the prospect chair."

The sponsor would be led into the dining room for a cup of coffee or something to eat and perhaps a quick tour of the house. Then, the sponsor would be invited to leave.

The prospect chair is a Daytop institution that goes back to the beginning and has been a part of the admission process ever since. It's a normal waiting-room chair, and it sits right in the front lobby of the Daytop Entry Unit. This is our "Grand Central Station," the busiest room in the place. Residents and staff members are coming and going in all directions. Groups are meeting and letting out. The phones never let up.

Sitting in the chair, amid all that activity, the newcomer gets a first glance at this frenetic and peculiar place. At the same time, Daytop is getting its first glimpse of the person in the chair. As the prospective resident is sitting in that busy lobby, a familiar face may pass by—perhaps someone from the old neighborhood, or an old customer or dealer from the drug business.

"Trevor!" the newcomer will say excitedly. Or, "Consuela! God, how have you been?"

But there is something odd about the interaction. The person in the chair will notice that no eye contact was made. The Daytop resident just kept on walking, pretending not to hear the newcomer speak. Even an outstretched hand will be ignored.

This is nothing personal. It's just a rule of the house. We don't yet know which way this new person is pulling—toward life or toward death. Until we discover the answer to that question, we really can't afford to get involved.

But these blank stares can be a little disconcerting. "This is a real nut house," the person in the chair might well be thinking by now. Or, "it's got to be some mind-control cult." Sitting there, the applicant may or may not have noticed that, despite all the weird behavior, the Daytop people do look vibrant and obviously alive.

There is something else the person probably didn't notice: that the director of the Daytop Entry Unit had been gathering some first impressions of her own.

The director will notice, for instance, whether the young person in the prospect chair is sitting comfortably or not. Remember what the Daytop staff member said in that last phone call yesterday: "You're off drugs as of right now."

So if the person is sitting there comfortably, if there's no obvious anxiety, no signs of drug withdrawal, then a fairly confident prediction can be made: The commitment from yesterday was broken. The caller used drugs after getting off the phone.

In that case, the person will be sitting on the prospect chair for a long, long time. It could be twelve hours before the newcomer is called in for an interview. And no one will be making much of a fuss as those hours tick by. No food. No conversation. At most, the person will be offered an occasional cigarette.

On the other hand, if the person in the prospect chair seems hyperactive and agitated, that's a sign that drug withdrawal already has begun. The no-drug commitment from yesterday was honored. The interview will begin right away.

I've sat through many prospect interviews over the years. Every one of them is a little bit different. They are conducted by a team of four or five Daytop residents and staff members, and each team does things its own special way. But two bases have to be touched. The prospective Daytop resident should be given some idea of how the program operates. And before anyone can be accepted into the Daytop family, that person must—genuinely and explicitly—ask for help.

It's that "investing-in-your-own-recovery" again.

I remember one day a few years ago, the State Department sent an official delegation from Bulgaria to visit Daytop. They were three government officials and a translator. I met them at two o'clock in the lobby of the Entry Unit and gave them my short version of what Daytop is.

Then, I asked the Entry Unit director whether anything special was going on that afternoon. She said a prospect interview was getting started shortly. Through the interpreter, I told the Bulgarians that this might give them a sense of what our work entails. Did they have time to sit in on the interview? They would be delighted to stay, they said.

The interview was in the building's rotunda, a chapellike room on the ground floor. It had stained glass and wall-to-wall carpet. That afternoon, it was dark except for a small arc of light on the far wall. There were five residents and staff members sitting on one side of a table. Facing them on a stool was a dark-haired nineteen-year-old girl. Her name was Joan, and she looked drawn and pale from too many nights of snorting cocaine. She was still quite an attractive young woman, though.

"Hi, Joan," one of the people at the table said. "You've come to Daytop. Tell us a little about yourself."

She began laying out the details of a life in turmoil. She was an only child, she said, from a middle-class suburban town in northern New Jersey. Her early childhood was as normal as could be.

Then, eight years ago, when she was eleven, her mother and father were killed in an airplane crash. She went on to describe several of the foster homes she bounced in and out of. She said she didn't get much love in any of them. So she responded like many young people do when they have no roots and no one to look after them. She acted out. She was arrested a few times. And the only way she knew how to block out the heartache and loneliness was to dive deeper and deeper into drugs.

That was the end of her narrative. There was a pause, and one of the staff members spoke. "All right, Joan, you've just told us you don't have anybody in the world. You've come to Daytop, and we care about you. We hardly know you, but that's what Daytop is, caring and love. That's how each of us came here. You have no one, Joan. Convince us that you need help."

She hesitated for a moment. But no one at the table was saying anything, so she spoke, quietly. "I need help," she said.

"If you really need help, cry out, 'Help me,' " one of the residents shot back. "You have no one else and you've had a pretty rough eight years since your mom and dad died."

"Help me," Joan said, slightly louder this time.

"Joan, we don't understand—we can't hear you," one of the Daytop residents said.

What they were trying to convey to her was that she was just verbalizing the call for help. It was lip service. She didn't really feel it.

This went back and forth two or three more times until one of the people at the table became so annoyed that he stood up and screamed at Joan: "You're not getting the message here. Follow with me now, Joan. Pretend you are in the North Atlantic. Your ship has hit an iceberg. Everyone has drowned. You are the only survivor. It's pretty damn cold in the water, and you are holding onto a log. It's the only thing that's keeping you above the water, this log. Joan, your life. I'm talking about your life. Your life is in real danger. Your legs are already freezing. They're numb. Hey, Joan, do you see what I see? There's a boat over there. You see that boat over there. Hey, Joan, it's death you're facing. Do you see that boat?"

Finally, the message sank through. Joan stood up and threw her arms open. She shrieked into the room: "Help me. Help me. Help me."

When the people at the table heard that message, that gnawing cry for help, they stood up and hugged Joan, tears in their own eyes.

"Congratulations," one of them said. "You are accepted into Daytop. You are our sister now."

They left the room with the new Daytop resident, and I turned to our visitors from Bulgaria. All through the interview, their translator had been whispering feverishly into their ears. I'm not exactly sure how much of the interview they followed. Apparently, they picked up the basic idea. They too were wiping tears from their eyes.

These prospect interviews are inevitably an emotional, moving scene. A drug addict, so fresh from the street, is screaming, "Help me. Help me. Help me." When this happens, we know that person is ready to try to change. We know, in fact, that treatment has already begun.

The prospect interview can take an hour. Sometimes it can take three. But when that breakthrough comes, the Daytop residents and staffers all jump up and rush over and hug the newcomer and say, "Welcome to our family."

The miracle that is Daytop is being passed on again.

ARRIVING, UNEASY AND UNSURE

8

> *The witch doctor succeeds for the same reason that all (physicians) succeed. Each patient carries his own doctor inside him. They come to us not knowing this truth. We are at our best when we give the doctor who resides within each patient a chance to work.*
>
> (Albert Schweitzer's answer to Norman Cousins when visiting him at his West African hospital and upon asking how anyone could expect to become better after being treated by a witch doctor.)
>
> —*Science Digest*, September 1981

At Daytop, we don't like to make a big deal out of the process of withdrawing physically from drugs. Of all the challenges an addict faces in treatment, physical withdrawal is one of the least difficult. In the months to come, far tougher battles will be fought over the mind and soul of the addict. But before we can get on to those things, the body must be separated from the drugs. In most cases, what this requires is time. Two or three days is usually enough.

It is, nevertheless, not an especially cheery two or three days. For years, drugs have been pumped into the body. Over time, the body has come to crave those drugs. Suddenly, the supply is yanked away, and so the body will react—with nausea, vomiting, fever, chills, soreness, headaches, and a rush of other symptoms.

That said, however, drug withdrawal is not nearly as wrenching an experience as people often say. Forget that melodramatic John Lennon song about going "Cold Turkey." Forget the drug-withdrawal horror stories you've seen in the movies and on TV. The myth has been blown way out of proportion. The reality of withdrawal is far from pleasant—but it isn't nearly as dreadful as the horror stories would have people believe. In fact, withdrawing from heroin or cocaine or most other street drugs is not much worse than getting through a bad case of the flu.

There are a couple of exceptions to this, depending on the exact drug or combination of drugs involved. Withdrawing from a methadone addiction, for instance, can be a truly alarming experience. That drug, which the government often gives to addicts as a substitute for heroin, takes such a hold of the user that sudden withdrawal can actually cause convulsions and death. Withdrawing from barbiturates can be just as bad. So when people addicted to those drugs show up at Daytop, we send them to a hospital, where they can withdraw under a doctor's care. But just about all the others—the heroin junkies, the crack addicts, the pill heads, the meth cookers, the PCP users, and all the rest, including the ones who mix and match whatever they can find—can withdraw right on the Daytop Entry Unit in Queens. Only the ones we think are too frail or who arrive addicted to some questionable drug will be referred to medical detoxification.

What those hyped-up scenes from the movies portray is an act that addicts have developed. It's a means of getting attention. In the hospital, if the addict screams loudly enough or trembles with sufficient drama, a nurse or a doctor will come rushing over, carrying a syringe. That's exactly what the addict is hoping for, a chemical to make the pain magically disappear. Similar playacting goes on when an addict withdraws in jail. The dramatic act is for the sake of macho image: "Look at him! He sure must have been a big-time heroin junkie." In the culture of the cellblock, that means he must also have been a big-time thief. Inmate status comes from things like that.

At Daytop, however, those theatrics do not fly. "Knock it off," the prospects are told firmly. They usually do.

"I had gone for one last, all-night crack-and-heroin binge right before I came into Daytop," recalled Marty, a nineteen-year-old

MONSIGNOR WILLIAM O'BRIEN

former skateboard champion who had moved from PCP to cocaine to crack. "I figured this could be my last chance to get high for a while." Marty had been arrested for what must have been the fifteenth time. Mostly, it was larcenies and burglaries and a few drug-possession charges. This latest time, however, he'd been caught with several hundred vials of crack. The judge agreed to give Marty one, final chance: Daytop or jail.

"The day before the appointment, I had sold some things from my brother's apartment, so I had money in my pocket," Marty said. "I knew the rule was that you couldn't bring any money with you into Daytop. So I told myself this meant I had to spend the entire wad—spend it getting high, you know."

Marty showed up on time for his 9:00 A.M. appointment at the Daytop Entry Unit. By midafternoon, he had gotten through the prospect interview, and he was feeling a little drained from that. He had been shown the room he would be sharing with four other Entry residents—his home for the next few weeks. He met two of his new roommates. One of them gave Marty a quick tour of the building and then started helping him put his clothes away.

About that time, Marty started feeling the first serious pangs of withdrawal.

Beads of sweat were forming on his forehead, and he noticed himself pacing around the room. He wiped his face off with one of his shirtsleeves. But the room was still feeling close. The roommate didn't need to be told why Marty was looking queasy. It was less than two weeks earlier that he had gone through precisely the same experience.

"I think I need something to drink," Marty said to the roommate. "Is there somewhere I can get some water around here?" He got directions to the water fountain, but something in the roommate's tone struck Marty as odd. "It was like he was saying, 'Okay, I'll tell you where it is.' But he wasn't expressing much sympathy for the way I felt. That's the clear impression I got."

The other residents in the Entry Unit are encouraged to go over and introduce themselves, stop by the new resident's room, maybe sit on the edge of the bed for a few minutes and chat. "I understand what you're going through—the physical and the mental things," they'll say. "Hang on. It's a little rough, but it's worth it. I was in the same place you are just a couple of weeks ago."

But we don't like to go too far with this. A little concern is fine. But when the newcomer starts with the overdramatic playacting, one of the other residents will come over and say: "Cut the crap. Leave those theatrics outside. Everyone here knows about withdrawing. We all made it through alive."

It will take the newcomer a while to understand this, but an important Daytop lesson is already being taught. We call this "acting as if." Act as if you know what you are doing. Before long, you really will know. Act as if you're not a baby. Before long, you won't be one anymore. Act as if you can handle the pain in life. Before long, you'll really be able to handle it. So we're not overly worried about a little fever and a headache. We don't pretend it's worse than it really is. We act as if we can handle it. Chances are, we can.

But Marty was just now getting his first inkling of this. At the same time, the fever was still hovering, and soon the nausea began to set in. He went back to his bedroom, and he lay down for a while.

Around dinner time, one of the Entry Unit counselors came by, and she sat down in a chair next to Marty's bed. "Marty," she said, "you remember during the prospect interview, the interviewers said your problem really wasn't drugs. Your problem was that you're a little baby locked into an adult's body.

"Well, the rule at Daytop is act as if you're a big boy. I know you're going through withdrawal. You're nauseated, and you're going to the bathroom all the time. Throwing up is never any fun, is it? But the rule of the house is to put something in your stomach at every meal. So why don't you put on your slippers and your bathrobe and go into the dining room with the rest of the family and have something to eat."

A terrible look rushed across Marty's face.

"I've thrown up three times already," he pleaded. "I really don't think I can keep anything down."

The counselor nodded understandingly, but she didn't back away. "Act like you're a big boy, Marty," she told him. "Do it anyway." In a few minutes, one of Marty's roommates came over and walked him down to the dining room. He didn't look very good. He was pale, and he was feeling dizzy. A couple of people in the hallway said hello to him. All Marty did was grunt.

Even after they got into the dining room, the roommate didn't let Marty sit down. Instead, he led Marty back into the kitchen and introduced him to a man in a white apron—the coordinator of the kitchen, the roommate explained.

"Good to meet you," the man in the apron said. He was tall and had a mustache. He had big gold fillings in several of his teeth.

"We love you and we're happy that you're our new brother," the kitchen coordinator told Marty. "In Daytop, you know, there's no free lunch. Why don't you come on in and wash a few dishes. That way, you can earn the right to sit down and put a little soup into your stomach."

Marty didn't know which sounded worse: standing in this industrial-sized kitchen washing dishes feeling like he did, or sitting down at a table and eating this man's soup.

His head was still spinning. He was still feeling queasy. But Marty did what the man told him to. He wasn't about to get a reputation for being a wimp this early in his time at Daytop. So he went over to the sink, and he squirted some detergent into a few glasses that were piled up there. When he got done with the glasses, one of the other kitchen workers brought over a big stack of bowls.

After a few minutes, the kitchen coordinator rescued Marty. "Okay, go on inside, my friend. Have a little split-pea soup."

Reluctantly, Marty filled a small bowl with the thick green liquid. He walked over to one of the tables and sat gently down. Slowly and methodically, he lifted two or three spoonfuls of soup into his mouth. He nibbled at the edge of a slice of white toast.

Before long, he was rushing off to the bathroom again.

It would take a while for Marty to appreciate what he went through that evening. It's not something many of our residents understand right away. But from the very first day at Daytop, a culture and an outlook are being instilled in the residents. Take responsibility for things. Work for what you get. Invest in your own recovery. That's the way people grow.

The idea is simple and old-fashioned, really. It's what the Entry counselor told Marty before she sent him down to eat. "Act as if." Your actions become internalized. Do the responsible thing. After a while, you become responsible. Without even realizing it, you'll grow into an adult.

On any given day, the Daytop Entry Unit has room for sixty-five men and women, all of them raw addicts just in off the street. This number doesn't include the teenage drug users who come to Daytop. They begin their treatment at our Adolescent Entry Unit in Rhinebeck, New York.

Adult Entry is located in Far Rockaway, a slightly down-on-its-heels neighborhood in the New York City borough of Queens. The Daytop center there is a block from the Atlantic Ocean and about an hour's ride by subway from Midtown Manhattan. This is the brand-new building that houses two other important arms of Daytop: the Pre-screen Unit, which handles admissions, and the Re-entry Unit, for Daytop residents who have completed the long-term treatment Upstate and are moving gradually back into society.

A typical stay on the Entry Unit could be anywhere from three to eight weeks, depending on how severe a human traffic jam we happen to have at the moment and how quickly a bed opens up in one of the houses Upstate.

Every morning, Daytop's Entry director, Donna Tannuzzo, makes a round of telephone calls known as the "bed count." "Anything open today?" Donna asks a staff member at each of the Upstate houses. "Anyone ready for Re-entry? Anybody split last night?"

This whole process works like a chain reaction. As a practical matter, someone has to complete the Upstate treatment—or drop out of Daytop completely—before someone down in Entry can be moved Upstate. And until that happens, there isn't room in Entry for the next addict to come in off the street.

This is the painful reality of limited resources. It is the great frustration we must live with every day. Twenty-one hundred young people fill our various centers. But the need outside is so tremendous. By comparison, we are so small. If anyone has a brilliant new answer to this depressing equation, I'd love to know what it is.

Entry, more than anything else, is a time for observation. It's a chance for us to get to know the people we have just invited to join our family and for them to get to know a little bit more about us. So right after arrival, each new resident is put through a battery of examinations—a full range of medical, psychiatric, and sociological tests. Daytop is not the solution for every addict's problems. We just don't have the facilities, say, to handle people with major medical problems. They have to go somewhere else first and get well. The same thing goes for people with severe psychiatric disorders. We're simply not equipped to treat such things. We refer these people to other programs that will better suit their needs. And for all concerned—us and them—it is better to discover these things before we waste too much of everybody's time.

Full-fledged treatment does not occur during Entry. The quarters are too cramped—and more importantly, the turnover is too swift—to match the intensity that is possible once these young people get to their houses Upstate.

At the same time, however, we don't want them just sitting around. The residents stay busy from early morning to late at night—a schedule they had better get used to if they are going to survive long at Daytop. Even if Entry cannot duplicate Upstate treatment, the new residents can be given a taste of what Daytop is all about.

They are introduced to concepts that, over the coming months, will begin to dominate their lives. Encounter groups. Seminars. Structured work assignments. The Daytop system of motivation and rewards.

And they start getting to know the members of Daytop's paraprofessional staff. These are mostly Daytop graduates, people who beat their own addictions with the help of these same techniques. Their work is augmented by professionals from the traditional disciplines—psychologists, social workers, physicians, and the like. But these Daytop-trained former addicts do the bulk of the hands-on work.

This, I believe, is one of the biggest reasons for Daytop's success. The personal histories of our staff generate immense credibility with residents—an I-have-been-there resume that can't be duplicated any other way. With it comes immeasurable patience and insight.

It is marvelous to watch the trusting relationships that this makes possible—between addicts who have conquered their addictions and those who have barely gotten through the door. Our counselors can tell what a youngster is feeling, or that a youngster is pretending, or when a youngster needs special help. That knack is not something that is taught in many graduate schools.

During those few weeks on the Entry Unit, we begin to instill the Daytop way of living into the confused and tormented minds of these sixty-five raw recruits.

One of the very first things we do is introduce the concept of discipline. Frequently, it's an utterly foreign concept. So we start out teaching the littlest examples of discipline. The new residents are shown how to make a bed, how to clean a room. They're shown how to clear tables, how to accept basic instructions, how to care for each other in extremely basic ways.

It is frightening to see how many of these supposedly sophisticated, worldly young people never even learned how to set a table.

The same way, the staff members work from the ground up on building the residents' social skills. "We have people coming together from all kinds of backgrounds," said James Robinson, a Daytop graduate who is the senior counselor on the Entry Unit. "We have all different races, different religions, different neighborhoods, different classes. For some of these people, Daytop is the first time they have ever been expected to interact maturely with people different from themselves."

So the residents are asked to stand up before the group and tell the others about themselves. "We work a lot on that," Robinson said. "The idea is that you are a guest here. Treat each other and treat Daytop with respect. Demonstrate that you have the ability to get along."

The new residents are introduced to "The Daytop Philosophy," a manifesto Daytop residents have been reciting since 1965. It was written by Richard Beauvais, a resident at the original Daytop house on Staten Island, who is now a college professor in Connecticut. The lines have already been translated into twenty-three languages around the world. A copy is on the wall in the dining room of the Entry Unit, and a version hangs somewhere at every Daytop facility there is. It goes like this:

> *I am here because there is no refuge,*
> *Finally, from myself.*
> *Until I confront myself in the eyes*
> *And hearts of others, I am running.*
> *Until I suffer them to share my secrets,*
> *I have no safety from them.*
> *Afraid to be known, I can know neither myself*
> *Nor any other; I will be alone.*
> *Where else but in our common ground,*
> *Can I find such a mirror?*
> *Here, together, I can at last appear*
> *Clearly to myself,*
> *Not as the giant of my dreams,*

Nor the dwarf of my fears,
But as a person, part of the whole,
With my share in its purpose.
In this ground, I can take root and grow,
Not alone anymore, as in death,
But alive, to myself and to others.

Those nineteen lines are about the closest thing we have at Daytop to a written manual for life. Residents on the Entry Unit are expected to learn them. In group meetings, the Philosophy is dissected line by line. It's used as a guide for meditation, a way of carefully reviewing the condition of one's life. Over the years it has proven to be a very useful tool.

Many new residents, when they first arrive at Daytop, are firmly convinced they will never get off drugs. Most of them have been using heavily for years. Many of them have tried to quit many times before and could never make it stick.

So they arrive at Daytop telling themselves, "I just need a little time to sit out the crisis of the moment," whatever it was that pushed them through the door. They look at Daytop as a place to hide awhile, rest up, get renourished, and return to a life of drugs.

This is not true of everyone, but the thought at least runs through the minds of most new Daytop residents. And we are not alarmed by it. We know that, at the beginning of treatment, all we have is the addict's body. It takes much longer to gain any meaningful influence over the addict's mind. But the seeds of future recovery are planted from day one.

The newcomers look around the Far Rockaway building, where the Entry Unit is. They also see the residents who are now in Reentry, the ones who have already made it through their treatment Upstate. Often, they will recognize some of these other residents from their own drug-using days. When they look at these people now, they seem strangely happy. Physically, they are healthy and their lives seem on track. This is bound to spark some interest.

This might sound like wonderful inspiration, and in a subtle way it is. But to a veteran user of street drugs, there's another possible interpretation, as well. "If these people are so happy and serene and together, they must be getting high. Surely, they're getting their drugs from somewhere. Maybe I'll wait around a little while, at least long enough to find out how to get drugs at Daytop." This is obviously a negative mindset, and frequently it lingers for a while.

We just keep on working, slowly subverting those negative assumptions by introducing the Daytop point of view.

Ever so slowly, almost imperceptibly at first, the new residents begin showing signs of understanding. Ever so slowly, they open their eyes to bigger possibilities. Ever so slowly, they start becoming the people they were pretending to be, the people they secretly wanted to be.

FINDING THE TOOLS FOR LIVING **9**

> *But one of the characteristics is that confrontations or encounters have to be done by people who are in the same boat. People are too fragile—Dr. Connell's patients are too fragile—for their defenses to be breached by doctors, social workers, ministers, parents, etc. These defenses can be breached and I don't think anybody is too fragile to have them breached, by relatively loving confrontation, by people who are in the same boat.*
>
> *Certainly my experiences with AA in observing half-way houses and in watching how relatively healthy people find ways of breaching the defensive detachment that Monsignor O'Brien refers to indicate that nobody is too fragile to have his defenses breached, if he is given enough social support and the encounter is done by peers and not by some deus ex machina psychiatrist.*
>
> **—George E. Vaillant, M.D.,**
> ***Drug Dependence: Treatment and Treatment Evaluation,***
> **Proceedings of Skandia International Symposia, Stockholm, 1975**

Just arriving Upstate can be a tremendous shock to the system of a hardened drug addict. To get by on the street, addicts are forced to learn an extraordinary set of survival skills: how to disguise their drug use, how to raise money fast, how to do business with an unsavory assortment of characters, how to dodge the law, how to manipulate the genuine concern of relatives and friends.

For someone trying to maintain a heavy addiction, these skills are almost essential. But in the highly structured world that Daytop creates, they are of no use at all. In fact, the drug-addict code of behavior is one of the most important things that Daytop works to change.

The real miracle of Daytop occurs at our eight residential treatment centers, which are in the rural foothills of the Berkshire and

Catskill mountains of Upstate New York. "Houses," these places are called in Daytop-speak. They are just a couple of hours from the crack houses and shooting galleries and street-corner drug markets of New York City, in a region of rolling hills and flat blue lakes. But for all the isolation of this idyllic landscape, it might as well be a million miles away.

The contrast is dramatic.

Five of the houses—one each in the small communities of Swan Lake, Parksville, and Nyack, two in Rhinebeck—are reserved for adults. The three other houses—one in Millbrook, two in Rhinebeck—are strictly for teenagers. All eight are run on the same basic principles. They are coed, and they include residents from every kind of background. For ten or twelve or fourteen months, one of these big, rambling houses becomes the addict's home. The people who live there—the staff and the other recovering addicts—become the new resident's family. And everyone in the household is working day and night toward the same life-saving goals: self-knowledge, maturity, honesty, caring, responsibility and, of course, victory over drug abuse.

"Schools for living," we call these Upstate houses.

The physical isolation is not by accident. We have discovered that a little distance from the tug of the city can be a useful thing. So Daytop plops its residents out in the country, far from old friends and old temptations, into a world where all the rules have changed.

Here, in the middle of nowhere, we can take the addict's street code and turn it on its head. In Daytop, the rules say: Be honest. Be open. Be responsible. Live by the law of the house. Work for what you get. Leave behind the self-destructive life of the addict— the hiding, the manipulation, the dishonesty, the eternal selfishness. Learn to be proud of yourself.

Daytop doesn't force drug addicts to change. No one can possibly do that. But we create a utopian world where fundamental change can occur. It is a world every bit as pressured as the old one, even more so in some respects. But the pressure now is pushing in a positive direction, toward life instead of death. By imposing this new set of rules and expectations, we begin rebuilding shattered lives.

Those few weeks on the Entry Unit in Queens were really just a prelude to the things that happen next. Entry was an important time of transition, a chance for the addict to ease in off the street, to be separated from the drug, to get vertical again. By the time the new resident arrives Upstate, the physical symptoms of withdrawal have passed. The urgency of addiction has subsided a little. That desperate sense of drowning is gone.

But compared to the new challenges the resident will find Upstate, those were relatively easy accomplishments. Mentally, the person is still very much a drug addict. The battle against psychological dependence has barely begun. And that is a far tougher challenge than simply purging the body of drugs. We are struggling for the addict's soul.

"When I first got to Swan Lake, I really didn't know what to make of the place," recalled Robin, a nineteen-year-old mother of two who had her kids taken away six months after she became addicted to crack. "I just remember thinking that the house seemed like a big mansion, with all these people hurrying all over the place."

(All eight of the Upstate houses have colorful histories. Swan Lake happens to have been a resort hotel, part of the legendary "Borscht Belt" where old-time stand-up comedians like Milton Berle, Henny Youngman, and Buddy Hackett got their starts. Rhinebeck's Fox Run Campus was once home to the great writers Thomas Wolfe and Aldous Huxley.)

"Back when I was in Entry, everybody was always saying, 'This is nothing. Just wait till you get Upstate.' I didn't know what they were talking about, and nobody could really explain it to me.

"One time, I asked one of the counselors down there. He tried to tell me a little bit. But basically, it just came down to him saying, 'You'll see.'

"My whole time on the way up in the van, I was trying to imagine where I was going to. I was thinking, 'This is a long way from the city.' That made me nervous. I was saying to myself, 'I'm not really the country-girl type.' "

But when she got there, Robin was struck mostly by the enormity of the house—and how busy everyone seemed.

"Everybody was walking in and out and up and down, all over the place," she said. "I didn't know what it was all about. People were going to their job assignments, probably. They were going to their encounter groups. They were doing all kinds of things. I was like, 'It's gonna take a little while for me to figure this place out.' "

Almost all of our residents come to Daytop from families I would call broken. By that, I don't just mean families where the mother and the father are separated or divorced—although we do get plenty of those. I mean broken in an even more important respect. These families failed to teach the children some of the basic skills of life.

This is disturbingly common today.

Had these young people learned to exercise responsibility, had they been taught the values of honesty and openness, had they developed discipline and self-control, they never would have taken refuge in the self-destructive world of drugs. Instead, they were passed some questionable values from their families. They compounded the problem with some even-worse values from the street. Then, they woke up one day and discovered their lives were an awful mess.

What Daytop does is re-create the family—and run the youngster through a second time. But now this family is a healthy one, a family with rules and expectations, a family built on this thing we call demanding love. It is that love that says, "I love you so much I refuse to baby you. I want you to grow and become responsible." It's not a sympathetic love or a love that says, "Don't worry because I'll protect you from anything bad that might happen." It's a love that has to be earned.

Each of the Daytop houses Upstate is run like a separate family. This is true in just about every sense of the word. Members of the Daytop staff serve as the authority figures. The residents are expected to treat one another like brothers and sisters. And everyone is in it together—sharing, caring, looking out. We even use the word without being bashful. "Good morning, family," a resident will say after standing up at Morning Meeting. Or, "Excuse me, family, there's something I have to say."

It might sound odd to outsiders. But the family we create Upstate has a strong, beautiful pull. It really has a way of changing lives.

Let there be no mistake about it: this is a family with rules. From the moment a new resident arrives Upstate, he or she is being indoctrinated into the culture of the Daytop house.

Rules are a powerful way of saying, "I love you." There are lots of rules at Daytop, and none of them is treated as trivial. But two rules are considered even more important than the rest.

No drugs.

No violence.

Break one of those cardinal rules, and in a hurry, you'll be shown the door.

On the street, these were the two primary ways—drugs and violence—that addicts dealt with stress. Childishly, the addict lashed out with violence. Or just as childishly, the addict ran away and hid from the problems of the moment with the aid of some mind-numbing drug.

"No drugs" at Daytop means even the smallest amount. No stashes in the bedroom. No stray pills in the pocket of a coat. And no drinking, either. Alcohol is just another drug, and Daytop must be kept completely drug free. Prescription medications—even aspirin—are closely regulated by the nursing staff. Our residents, remember, are people who not long ago did terrible damage to their lives with drugs. Even the tiniest step backward cannot be allowed.

Finding someone with drugs at Daytop is, thankfully, a relatively rare occurrence. It is a fundamental violation of the reason the resident is here, and it represents a threat to the strides that other residents have made. So when it happens, we have to respond harshly. We send the person home. Someone who holds on to drugs at Daytop is not ready to be serious about life.

Violence in the house is treated in much the same manner—and for many of the same reasons—as drugs.

In the street-addict's culture, threats and violence were the easy ways of achieving difficult goals. "I want something you have, so I'll beat you up to get it." Or, "You moved onto my drug-selling territory, so I'll shoot you." Or "You and I have a disagreement—even a little disagreement—and we'll settle it the macho way, with our fists, our knives, or our guns."

When we say violence at Daytop, we mean any sort of physical confrontation, between two residents or between a resident and a member of the staff. We also mean verbal or other kinds of threats. All of it is unacceptable inside the family.

At Daytop, the goal is to get beyond these childish ways of confronting stress—lashing out or running away—and replace them with something more healthy and mature.

Beyond the two cardinal prohibitions, Daytop residents are expected to follow a whole panoply of other rules. Some of these are based on common courtesy. Some of them are made necessary by the logistics of so many people in one house. And some of them are designed to teach special lessons that many of the residents failed to learn when they were living outside.

From the moment a new resident arrives at Daytop, these norms of drug-free living are being taught.

The residents are expected to work hard and have pride in their work. They are taught not to take anything that isn't theirs. "Borrowing" without asking is considered stealing at Daytop—one of many ways in which the amoral code of the street is reversed. They are told never to make assumptions about things they don't understand at Daytop. If in doubt, ask.

The residents are supposed to treat each other like siblings and always show "responsible concern." This means do what is good for the other resident, even if it conflicts with what the person wants.

"Pull in" the younger brothers and sisters, the residents are taught. Help them learn the norms of life at Daytop. And don't subscribe to the "see-no-evil" code of the street. If someone is violating the trust of Daytop, help that person and help the family by getting involved. This is part of the art of showing responsible concern.

Be honest. Be open. Be self-reflective. Daytop is not a place for secrets. Only through openness and frankness will there be growth. And no "negative contracts," agreements between residents to cover for each other.

Confront other residents. "Get out on the floor," in the house's common areas. Don't spend too much time alone. Isolation can inhibit growth. The other residents are brothers or sisters. Flirting or sex inside the family is considered taboo. Daytop residents have serious business before them. This is not the time to be starting sexual relationships. (Sex, we tell the residents, is a gift shared between two people. During treatment, this is not a gift you have to give. First, you must re-create yourself as a person. Until that's been accomplished, you are not ready for a relationship. Someday, you will be. Then, it will be meaningful and beautiful.)

Orders from staff members and from senior residents in positions of authority must be followed without question. Protesting or objecting or even grumbling about a direction is not okay. It is fine to feel bad or be angry. But the residents are expected to learn control over these things.

Such feelings are not to be ignored. They are to be channeled and dealt with in a mature, reasonable fashion. One of the big problems the addict faced out on the street was an inability to get along in a structured environment. It's something we're constantly working on Upstate.

That's a lot of rules.

To an outsider, the sheer volume might seem oppressive. And in a sense, it is. But we are trying to deal with some intransigent, deep-seated problems here. We need to break a group of hard-core drug addicts of the norms they've lived by for years. Even if the desire to change is there, these old patterns die hard. Laissez-faire simply will not do the trick.

So we have created a world that is heavily structured. Success and failure are clearly defined. An easy-to-understand hierarchy is established. Rewards and punishment are clear.

It's true, we demand a high degree of conformity. But before our residents can learn to exercise independent responsibility, they have to learn to live by someone else's rules.

The days Upstate are long, and the residents are kept busy all day. Somehow or other, though, every part of the daily schedule is designed to further treatment—even the things which might not seem like that at first.

Everyone gets up at seven o'clock in the morning. Rooms are straightened. Beds are made military style. Breakfast begins in the communal dining room at seven thirty. By nine, the day's activities have begun.

Meetings. Discussion groups. Seminars. Encounter groups. Class work. Job training. Therapy sessions. They are scheduled all through the day and into the evening. And that's not all. For two hours in the morning and two and a half hours in the afternoon, the residents are assigned specific job functions around the house. This allows the houses to operate with relatively few outside employees. And it gives the residents a chance to learn—often for the first time—the skills and the satisfactions of work.

The days stay full. A year or so of Upstate treatment might sound like an eternity to a drug addict coming in off the street. But to remake a human being, it's a very short time.

The business of each day Upstate begins with Morning Meeting. Breakfast is over. The dishes are done. The residents' bedrooms should be tidy and clean. Everyone assembles in the dining room, ready to go by nine.

A staff member stands before the group, usually holding a clipboard.

"Good morning, family," the staffer says.

"Good morning, Paul," or "Good morning, Marilyn," the residents answer back.

The staff member welcomes everyone to the new day at Daytop, perhaps singling out a few residents with light questions about something that happened at breakfast or the night before, maybe asking how someone slept.

The staff member calls on someone to lead the group in reciting "The Daytop Philosophy." Then, the staff member runs through the schedule for the day, making sure to mention anything unusual that is planned. Any guests in the house are introduced. The residents are reminded about field trips and other special activities.

Finally, the floor is opened up for a formal round of "pull ups."

Outsiders are often shocked when they hear what a big deal we make of things most people would consider trivial. An ashtray with a few cigarette butts left sitting on a table. A light left on in an empty room. These breaches may seem minor in the outside world. But at Daytop they are of the utmost importance. They connote a non-caring attitude, a reversion to the old habits of the street. These are important tools for learning, and that's what "pull ups" are all about.

"Good morning, family," someone will stand up and say during the morning meeting.

"Good morning, Frank," the others answer in unison.

And then Frank points out some violation of the Daytop rules he noticed, or some insensitivity on someone's part. "Who is the person who left a half-empty coffee cup sitting on the window sill in the front hall. It was there about eight thirty last night, and when I found it, the coffee was already cold. So it must have been there for a while. I picked it up and brought it into the kitchen. But why would someone disrespect the house and family like that? Why should I be cleaning up for someone else?"

For a moment, the room might be silent. But almost always, someone will speak up.

"It must have been me," Celeste stands up and says. "After dinner, I was talking to Gregory in the living room. And he told me he would help me with an article I am trying to write for the paper. So we went into the living room. I might have forgotten to pick up the coffee cup."

"Might have forgotten?" the staffer asks.

"Well, more than 'might,' " she says. "I did."

"What do you learn from this?" the staffer asks.

"To be more careful. To respect the family's home. To stay in control of my possessions. Not to rush off places without thinking."

"Good. Anything else?"

"No, I can't think of anything."

"Anything else?"

"Oh yeah. I'm sorry, family."

"All right. Sit down."

Now, on its own, that stray coffee cup is not especially significant. But at Daytop, these things mean a lot. They are ways to teach lessons about responsibility, to get people to think about themselves.

Making a big deal of these things tells us that we care. So it's refreshing to see when the family is asked about an ashtray or a coffee mug, and a person raises his or her hand and says, "Yes, I did it. I'm sorry."

The utter honesty of Daytop can be jarring to an outsider. But to the young person coming up, strangely it can be almost a relief. It's the first time the new resident doesn't have to keep track of who's been told what lie and who'll be the one to squeal. At Daytop, the residents can afford to be totally honest. The honesty will be accepted and encouraged and welcomed, even if sometimes it comes with a price. Over time, the resident will learn that the price is more than worth it. And in return, the Daytop family will give the resident a huge supply of love.

Every Upstate resident has a daily job assignment, one of the many chores that must get done if the house is to function well. The assignment might involve staffing the telephone switchboard or working on the maintenance crew or driving one of the vans or—in the case of senior residents—actually helping the staff coordinate the treatment program.

These jobs are not distributed at random. New residents start at the bottom. The lowliest, most awful jobs, the ones with the lowest status and responsibility, are reserved for them. Frequently, newcomers are aghast when they arrive Upstate and discover what jobs are assigned to them: scrubbing pots and pans after meals, cleaning out toilets, doing heavy yard work in the summer, shoveling snow in the winter.

"I couldn't believe it," said Mark, a thirty-three-year-old cocaine addict who was one of the most successful drug dealers in Daytona Beach, Florida. "Two months ago, I was riding around in a Mercedes. I was doing $30,000 deals, buying and selling heavy weight."

The day after Mark arrived at the Daytop house in Parksville, he was handed a Brillo pad and pointed toward the kitchen sink. "You can't imagine how that feels. I was like, 'Dishes? You want me to wash dishes? I don't wash dishes.' I didn't say that. But that's what I was thinking."

The kitchen coordinator did not seem interested in negotiating, and Mark got to work on a big iron stew pot.

None of these tasks is glamorous. But we insist that all the Daytop houses be immaculately kept. So every job must be done. These work assignments are one of the ways the residents at Daytop learn to change their lives.

The work assignments are built around a simple system of status and reward. Do well on pots and pans, and you'll move up to plates and dishes. Keep doing well, and you'll get out of the kitchen entirely. Screw up, and even more quickly you'll be bounced back down.

The goal is to get residents to work hard and exercise responsibility—and take pride in their work. Step by step, the residents learn to climb the ladder of success. Only by performing well at the bottom, do the more interesting, more challenging, more prestigious possibilities at the top open up. After a while, the person even begins to see real meaning in cleaning toilets well or scrubbing pots and pans well. The resident learns that progress begins at the bottom. Only by accepting responsibilities and working hard can success ever be achieved. Slowly but almost inevitably, the person's outlook begins to change.

All this is little more than the old-fashioned Protestant work ethic. To outsiders, the system might seem almost pedestrian in its simplicity. But to someone who has spent years chasing after the quick thrills of drug use, the concept can seem like it comes from another world.

Work assignments—like so much else at Daytop—are set up along tightly drawn lines. The family is divided into work teams, each of which takes care of certain jobs. There are separate teams for the kitchen, for building maintenance, for the commissary, for procurement, and for something we call "expediting." Expediters are the residents who run errands and coordinate among the different teams.

Each team has its own internal system of power and responsibility. There are coordinators, assistant coordinators, foremen, and so on down the line.

The top jobs, of course, go to senior residents with proven leadership abilities. The lowest-status positions are assigned to the newcomers—or to more senior residents in need of remedial "learning experiences."

This system takes advantage of the normal human desire to strive for success. To that, it adds the pressure to become a "role model" for those below and the genuine pride most people feel in a job well done. The lessons here are not subtle: Do well, and you are rewarded. Do well long enough, and there is nothing you cannot attain.

At the same time these lessons are being taught through the work assignments, they are being reinforced inside the nightly meetings of the Daytop encounter groups.

Encounter groups at Daytop are different from the kind of group therapy that many people know. We don't tiptoe around each other's psyches, and we don't make secret deals to leave each other alone.

That's what often happens in the so-called encounter groups that have begun to spring up in some mental hospitals and penitentiaries across America. "Don't expose me, and I won't expose you," the participants promise each other. "That way, neither of us gets rattled. We'll both get through this thing unscathed."

Frequently, these deals are never spoken. But they are perfectly understood. The therapy sessions remain gentle and pleasant. No one's attitudes are ever threatened. No one is challenged by anyone else. And of course, no one learns anything.

Encounter groups at Daytop are anything but gentle. They are loud and vulgar. They are raucous and rough. All emotions are considered legitimate. No one's feelings are spared. The sessions get so intense sometimes, they are painful even to sit through. At Daytop, when we say frank and open exchange, that's exactly what we mean. And nowhere is its form as pure as in the regular encounter groups.

Just walk through the house when the groups are meeting. Through the open doorways, you will hear all sorts of supercharged complaints.

"You dis'ed me, Myron," a young woman is screaming, in a blood-curdling tone. "I liked you. I thought you were my friend. Then, I find out you're talking about me to Yvette. You're making fun of my red sweater, saying I look stupid when I wear it, saying that hood it has on the back looks queer. How could you do that? I trusted you. I thought you were my friend. Now, you make me feel stupid. You took advantage of my friendship. That's what you did. How could you do that to me?"

The young woman, whose name was Concetta, went on like this for another minute or so. Finally, in a much softer voice, Myron spoke up. He acknowledged that he shouldn't have made the crack about Concetta's sweater. It's a perfectly nice sweater, he said. But, he continued, he was angry about her leaving early from their joint work assignment the previous afternoon. That's why he was lashing out.

"How do you think that made me feel?" he asked. "Me staying there working like some fuckin' chump. You going off to hang around with your friends?"

"It's still no excuse," she shot back.

The sweater-and-the-duck-out-early matter will be resolved easily. And in other rooms around the house, other groups are dealing with similar feelings, hashing them out in much the same way.

The groups meet several nights a week, usually for two hours after dinner. The routine works like this: A shoe box is left out on a table in the dining room. Whenever a resident has a problem with someone else in the house, the resident writes both their names on a small piece of paper and puts the paper into the box.

This is called "dropping a slip" on someone.

Right before the next time the encounter groups are scheduled, a staff member sits down with the shoe box and divides the house into groups.

Each group has between ten and twelve residents and is led by a member of the staff. Every effort is made to match up the family members who have dropped slips on each other, and the groups are also generally balanced by race, sex, age, personality type, and other factors. Every time, the composition of the groups changes. So over the course of a few weeks, everyone should get into a group with just about everyone else.

At Daytop, the encounter group is the emotional safety valve. It's our way of diffusing bad feelings and making sure that violence doesn't break out.

Have hard feelings for someone in the family. Learn to channel those feelings. Learn a little self-control. The junkie's response would be to explode swiftly into violence or, perhaps, to run away. Neither of those is an acceptable response at Daytop.

Just about anything goes in group. There are only a few basic rules. No violence or threats of violence, of course. And the purpose is expression, not browbeating. So a little repetition is permitted. But the group leader will step in if the same thing is being said over and over again.

The leader focuses discussion on the daily lives of the people in the group—not on deeper speculation about why these people are as they are. The goal is to provide a "gut" experience, not self-defense or self-justification.

The language can be profane or vulgar. (At other times, talk like that is not tolerated at Daytop. In fact, vulgarity to another family member can be cause for "dropping a slip" on someone and confronting that person during group.)

And no one is immune. The encounter group is an utterly democratic institution. Everyone in the group is fair game for criticism, including staff members. Frank expression is expected. The goal is "constructive confrontation." Most of us shy away from these kinds of encounters in our lives. We tell ourselves it is safer not to get involved. If I criticize someone else, they might criticize me.

But in group at Daytop, honesty, even the most painful kind, is expected from all. The exchange can be provocative. But the petty disagreements of the day are faced inside the group. And they don't fester and grow into larger problems. They are dealt with in a healthy way.

Sometimes, the experience of the encounter group—no matter how well executed—just isn't enough. So we have developed a variety of special groups to take care of special needs.

There are peer groups for people who came to Daytop at about the same time. This is one way for people dealing with some of the same personal issues to gain strength from one another. It also helps build a special peer-group camaraderie.

There are static groups. There are feelings groups. There are groups set up around almost any need.

And there are groups that run on for hours and hours. They produce a level of intensity that is almost impossible to achieve in the usual hour or two. These include what we call extended groups, which run for as long as eighteen continuous hours, and marathons, which go round the clock for three or four days. In the marathon, the residents are expected to dig some very painful incidents from their childhoods, feelings that were long since buried. These memories come rushing forward in outbursts of hurt and tears. That's when you're really getting down to the bedrock of human feelings.

These extended groups and marathons aren't held often—perhaps two or three times during a resident's stay Upstate. But they are the "power tools" of the Daytop treatment program.

Usually, the extended groups are built around a particular theme—often something that has grown into an issue of some kind around the house. Prejudice might be the topic, or competition or self-control.

The marathons, the most intense of all, are as draining and as useful as group encounters can be. More free form than the extended groups, marathons are designed to help the residents work through four problem areas that almost everybody has: expressing and accepting anger, giving and receiving love.

There's almost nothing that's not dug up in one of these marathon sessions. Sharing such deep feelings produces a beautiful bonding among the group members. At Daytop, the people who went through a marathon together are often closer to one another than to anybody else.

• • •

Some drug addicts can be very charismatic. Out on the street, they rely heavily on their ability to charm and manipulate others, essential techniques in the constant quest for drugs. Most addicts, however, are not nearly so glib. They are shy. They lack self-confidence. Or having spent all that energy chasing after drugs, they simply never developed strong social skills. Frequently, the deeper an addict sinks into drug use, the more severe this interpersonal discomfort becomes.

That is something else we work on at Daytop. It's what the daily seminars are all about.

Most weekday afternoons, from one to two o'clock, all the residents in the house gather in the dining room. One of the staff members gets things started by taking a piece of chalk and writing a sentence or a paragraph on the board.

It's usually an intellectual idea—something from literature or philosophy or history or the social sciences. Then, the floor is open to all. The idea is for this roomful of addicts to see the possibility of cultural exchange.

The topic of the day could be a brief passage from James Baldwin. It might be one of the Ten Commandments, or a slogan from a TV ad. Some days, it's an out-of-the-blue statement like, "Fire is more powerful than water." Other days, it could be a nursery rhyme.

The specific topic isn't really important. The point is to get people to think abstractly and to learn to express themselves. The brain, after all, is like a muscle. To stay strong, it has to be exercised. So in seminar, everyone is urged to join in.

To the new residents, these after-lunch meetings can seem puzzling at first. "I remember thinking the first few times I went to seminar, 'Who cares about some sentence from Anaïs Nin?'" recalled Paco, a heavy-set boy whose main form of expression on the street was the grunt. "Who cares about the Japanese competitiveness? Who cares about what Copernicus thought? Don't I have big enough problems on my own?"

Many residents are reluctant to speak up in the beginning. They are bashful about expressing themselves. So they'll sit there and listen to others. And slowly, their confidence will build. After a relatively short time, they will stand up and be heard.

"So much of this problem with the Japanese," Paco was saying one day during his third week Upstate, "is in the mind of the Americans. We've gotten ourselves into feeling inferior. We've stopped believing in ourselves. We do that for very long and after a while, of course we'll produce worse cars. And the whole thing will just get worse from there."

"That's only part of it," a young woman named Sandra piped in. "They cooperate more with each other, and they work harder than we do."

"We're the ones who are to blame," said another woman on the other side of the room. "We're the ones who buy their cars and their TVs. We're not supporting our own industries. That's why so many Americans are out of work."

Is Paco right about that? Maybe he is. Maybe he's not. On this particular afternoon, the other residents who spoke during the seminar came down on various sides. That's not the point. What's important is to get people comfortable with expressing themselves.

Soon, they are standing on their feet and giving their thoughts on complicated subjects.

They learn to express themselves, to stake out a position, to explain their thoughts to a group, to defend something they believe.

A roomful of drug addicts engaged in these complex philosophical discussions. It's really something to see.

There is no set timetable for how quickly someone should complete treatment Upstate.

Different people learn to change their lives at different paces. "Putting in the time"—that basic currency of the jailhouse—does not measure progress at Daytop. Progress comes only with personal growth.

Thankfully, most residents do progress. They gain confidence from their own successes. They are lured by the promise of greater status and more responsibility. They are attracted by the examples the older residents set. Over time, they decide they like themselves better as they move far beyond the drugs.

But this comes slowly. At every step of the way, the residents have to prove themselves. That's what demanding love is all about.

The residents learn to submit to the regimen of the house. They learn to delay the response to the wants they feel. They learn to care about one another. They learn to be trusting, believing, brutally honest. This is something I warn first-time Daytop visitors about: "Don't ask one of our kids 'How are you?' unless you're ready to hear the answer. You could be standing there for a while."

All these changes are going on. But the main change is to integrate values that are the reverse of the values on the street. When we describe ourselves as a "School for Living," this is what we mean.

First of all, the residents learn that they can no longer use people the way they used to. They can no longer con the people who care about them. Instead, they learn, they must be totally honest. There is no substitution for that.

Second, they discover that honesty demands a hard look in the mirror and some deep thought about their place in the future. For the first time ever, this will make the addict love himself, or consider herself truly worthwhile.

And third, Daytop residents come to understand the message, "There is no free lunch." Love demands a price, and every step of progress must be earned. So must every privilege. Whether it's writing home or telephoning or having visits—going right up the scale to the point where the resident is ready for Re-entry—the hierarchy of responsibilities must be climbed.

What's left are the lessons about how to take all this caring and responsibility out into the world.

This requires an honest and positive style of living. And it requires understanding a paradox that is not always easy to understand. The paradox is this: You cannot keep what you have taken from your Daytop experience unless you keep giving it away.

That's the credo for the outside. In the months that follow, Daytop residents learn to practice that important paradox in their increasingly independent lives.

THE ROAD BACK **10**

Drugs do not cause addiction! Alcohol does not cause alcoholism! As long as we still labor under the most primitive, uncritical and unscientific impression that an inert substance is capable of generating a phenomenon like 'addiction,' as long as we pay homage to this theory . . . we will never understand what the phenomenon of 'addiction' and, especially, 'alcoholism,' could teach us about coping with life, dealing with conflict or structuring or managing life.

—Walther H. Lechler, M.D., 1991 Symposium,
Promethean Institute, Milford, Pennsylvania

Re-entry is the make-or-break stage of treatment. It is the most delicate and crucial part of everything Daytop does.

For a recovering addict, the drugs used to provide a curtain that could be pulled down against pain. The drugs filled a vacuum in the addict's life and helped disguise the core of emptiness most of us occasionally feel inside. During that year or so Upstate, Daytop ripped back the curtain and let some light shine in. It filled the vacuum where the drugs once were and equipped the addict with some coping skills that turn out to be far more useful than the drugs. The result is a splendid, maturing adult.

But Daytop's work isn't over yet—with a quick "goodbye" and "good luck."

After what goes on Upstate, you can't just plop these young people back out on the street. You have to ease them out of treatment. And the return must be gradual, strategic, and monitored carefully every inch of the way—the same way an experienced scuba diver returns from the deep. The cocoon of Daytop is opened slowly. And at the first sign of trouble, we have to be there to lend support.

"I was Upstate for a little more than a year, working harder than

I had ever worked at anything before, trying to rebuild my life," said Neil, a thirty-one-year-old heroin addict from a big Italian family in Bensonhurst, Brooklyn. Neil had been one of our most impressive Upstate residents. He had a loud, booming laugh, and he always took the time to look out for the younger family members. But even though Upstate treatment had gone relatively smoothly for him, Neil discovered that this didn't mean Re-entry would be a breeze.

"For the first time ever, I was becoming really confident with myself," Neil recalled. "I was really excited about coming back to the city. But no matter how you look at it, Upstate is an artificial world. I had never tested my confidence on the outside. And to be honest, I was scared. I hadn't lived a straight life for, like, fifteen years. I had never held what you would call a normal job. And it wasn't like I had this great resume I could pass around."

Re-entry can take anywhere from six months to a year, and the process is divided into three phases; Re-entry A, B, and C. With each new phase, the residents achieve more independence. Little by little, the outside world is allowed to intrude.

We warn the residents how difficult this process can be, even before they move out of the house Upstate. "You'll be going back into the world where you once used drugs," we remind them. "It's up to you to confront that world in a healthier way. Daytop will be there for you. But it's not the same thing as living with your family Upstate. You won't have that placid environment, or all that security and support. You'll have to take all those things you learned Upstate and apply them in this harsher world. Constantly, you'll have to challenge that world with your newly ingrained openness, honesty, maturity, responsibility and caring."

This is what it means, finally, to be grown up.

The truth of it is that the residents get an eyeful of that new world the minute they arrive at Re-entry. The Re-entry Unit is located at the big Daytop center in Far Rockaway, Queens, the same building where the Entry Unit is. So the culture of the street is never far away. The phones are ringing constantly with drug addicts looking for a place to land. Prospective residents are coming in for their Pre-screen interviews. And the wide-eyed rookies on the Entry Unit are struggling to get adjusted to their new lives inside. Some of them are still going through the pangs of physical withdrawal.

It is a jarring contrast to the bucolic life Upstate.

At least, that's how Neil felt when he got back to New York. "It was like you'd lived your whole life in a small town somewhere," Neil said. "And you'd never left that small town. Then, you took a train one day and got off at Grand Central Station. There were all these people there, and all these lights and activity. In a way it was exciting. But in another way it was also scary."

During the first phase of Re-entry, the residents live and work at the Daytop center in Queens. But most of their energy is devoted to preparing for the practical realities of moving out. This might mean taking one last vocational course or finishing up some schoolwork. The Daytop staff and a cadre of outside volunteers teach a special series of classes on job hunting, money management, personal poise, and other useful skills.

At the same time, the Re-entry residents are also expected to help run the building. And they continue to get together for frequent seminars and encounter groups and other sessions like the ones Upstate. Re-entry is a rough time for most people. If they don't remain honest with themselves and open with the others in the group, their chances of success are not very bright. There are too many forces pulling in the other direction.

"The hardest thing about Re-entry is keeping your balance," said Dana, a tiny, blond-haired girl who was just sixteen when she came into treatment. She looked even younger than that a year and a half later, when she reached the Re-entry phase. "You still have the security of your family, the Daytop people. But they used to be the only factor there. You're still around them all the time. But in Re-entry, all these other factors start coming in, too."

Sometimes, conflicts arise. "It's like there are two different worlds," she said. "You have your friends and your real family and the other people you know. And you have Daytop. What you have to do is take the things you learned in Daytop and apply them back here. They're good lessons. You have to make them work for you, as you move out of here."

With the final two phases of Re-entry—B and C—the residents move gradually out on their own.

During Re-entry B, residents live at Daytop but spend their days outside. For most people, this means getting a job or returning to school full time. They're still sleeping at Daytop, still brushing up on the practical skills of independent living and still attending group meetings in the evening. But they are making their own money and saving for the day they'll move completely out of the house.

That comes in the final phase of treatment before graduation, Re-entry C. The resident moves out of the Re-entry House and into an apartment on the outside, perhaps with another Daytop person at first.

People at this stage of treatment still come back for group meetings in the evening—twice a week at first, once a week later on. And Daytop is still there to help in times of crisis. But their recovery has reached the point that a healthy, stable life outside is possible— often for the first time in many years.

At Daytop, Re-entry is the stress house. We manufacture stress and purposely impose it on the residents. This isn't done out of spite. It's our way of discovering how well they grew during Upstate treatment and how well they've learned to deal with the more conventional difficulties of day-to-day life.

Remember, most drug addicts have great trouble handling stress. That's a big reason many of them turned to drugs in the first place. Life grew stressful—as it does for everyone—and their answer was to self-medicate. During those months Upstate, they were supposed to have been learning more mature answers. So from time to time during Re-entry, we turn up the heat a little and see how they do. Frequently, the results are painful.

I remember one Friday night when I was leaving the headquarters building on Fortieth Street. An adorable boy named Timmy was working the front desk. That desk is staffed twenty-four hours a day. It's one of the work assignments the residents in Re-entry A are responsible for.

As I came out of the elevator, I said hello to Timmy. In typical Daytop fashion, he and I didn't shake hands. We gave each other a hug.

"Timmy, I love you," I said.

"I love you, too," he answered. That's when I noticed he was crying.

"What's the problem, Timmy?" I asked him. And he told me a story.

"You know," he said, "when I used drugs, my self-worth was minus zero. I remember back then, there was this girl I really liked, and I wanted to go out with her. But I never could get up the courage to ask her out on a date. Now I understand that was because I couldn't handle the rejection. I really didn't like myself.

"The girls I did go around with were not really people I cared about. It was stupid. We were shooting drugs together. We were killing each other. Now, since I've been at Daytop, I've learned that I am a good person, that I can achieve in life. I'm proud of what I've done so far. I know I'm going to be proud of everything I do from now on, and I'm going to be totally honest with myself and other people."

I wondered what Timmy was driving at. Then, he got to the point. "There's this great girl that I met," he said. "She's wonderful. And it's scary, you know. She knows everything about me, and she still loves me. I told her my whole story—how I messed up my life and everything—and she says she loves me, in spite of all that."

Timmy said he had just gotten his first permission for a weekend out of the house. "This was going to be our big weekend together," he said. But that afternoon, just as he was putting his clothes in his overnight bag, one of the counselors broke the bad news. Timmy's permission had been revoked. No explanation. No apology. Just canceled, like that.

"I really care about this girl," Timmy said to me, his eyes welling up again with tears. "I've been doing great in Re-entry. I deserve the permission. There was no reason for them to do that. It's totally unfair."

I could understand perfectly well how Timmy felt. Anyone in his position would feel exactly the same. But I tried to explain to him why it is so important that he learn how to deal with setbacks like this.

"You remember those themes that are up on the wall in Parksville?" I asked him. "Remember one of them says, 'Trust your environment'? Well, you have to trust it. Trust your environment."

Timmy looked at me like I was crazy, like I had completely missed the point of what he had just said.

What Timmy didn't know was that on Monday night, when he went into his group, they were going to say to him, "Timmy, how did it feel to have that permission pulled?"

Chances are, Timmy would break down crying again, and he would tell the others how much it hurt. He would explain how angry it made him and how foolish he felt when he had to tell his girlfriend that their weekend plans were off.

Finally, one of the counselors would explain. "We did that deliberately, Timmy, because in life, things like that happen. You have to learn to handle them. No, it's not fair. It's not right. But that's life. The question is, What are you going to do? Are you going to go back to drugs? Are you going to hurt yourself again when others hurt you? Are you going off in search of some new crutch? Or are you going to be smart and responsible? Learn from the pain and do your best to turn it around?"

It's a hard lesson but an important one. In the end, I think, Timmy learned it well. And the following weekend, he got that permission, which he certainly deserved. His girlfriend understood, and eventually even Timmy did, too. No pain. No gain. Last time I talked to him, Timmy was still doing great. He was working for an export company and living without drugs. He and the girlfriend were talking about getting married.

All through treatment, these young people have been learning how to live honest, caring, drug-free lives. They learned the importance of never compromising those fundamental values. They were taught to be role models and change agents out in the world.

Then, they get outside. The world out there, they discover, is not the loving and supportive place that they knew Upstate. It can be harsh and dishonest. It includes people whose values are going to clash with the ones Daytop taught. Compromise, many people say. Do the easy thing. Give in. Get high. Don't work so hard.

"The world is not a utopian place," we tell the Daytop kids. "You'll have to learn to deal with this. You can choose your friends carefully. You can stay away from people who use alcohol and drugs. You can surround yourself with a circle of nurturing and support. But in the end, you cannot hide from all the bad things in the world."

The trick is to take the lessons learned Upstate and apply them to the outside world. "Face these challenges openly and honestly," we say. "You've been given the foundation to do that."

That's what Suzie found when she was in Re-entry B. Suzie was a very athletic young woman. She had been an All-Conference girls' basketball player in high school—before she discovered cocaine. And even well into her drug use, she was still running marathons.

Eventually, the drugs took their toll on her body. When Suzie first showed up at Daytop, she could hardly walk, much less run. But after fourteen months of hearty eating and workouts in the Swan Lake gym, she arrived in Re-entry in tip-top shape.

When it came time for her to get a job, she decided she was interested in the exercise field. She arranged an interview at a health club and they offered her a trainer's job right away.

She loved the job, and the club members she worked with thought she was terrific. She had been there about three months, when she came into my office one day. She was obviously upset.

"Why the tears?" I asked her.

The problem was her job, she said. "I like the work and everything," she said. "The clients are nice. You know I love being around sports all day. But something happened yesterday, and it was just awful."

I asked her to explain.

"There's a lady who comes to the club named Mrs. Rawls. She's been coming for a couple of months. She's a little heavy, and she wants to lose some weight. I don't know what the problem is, but she's not losing at all."

Apparently, Mrs. Rawls had complained the day before to the health-club manager, and the manager had spoken to Suzie about the situation. "He told me I'm supposed to adjust the scale in a certain way, so she'll think she's losing weight," Suzie said.

"The first time, I did lie to her," Suzie said. "But I couldn't handle the lie. I felt so guilty. The second time, I refused to do it. I just didn't tell her anything. That was this morning, and I had to come over and talk with you."

I looked at her sitting there. "Suzie," I said, "I love you. But you're going to have to quit that job. There's no compromise on this one, I'm afraid."

"I'm so glad you said that," she told me, beaming now. "I couldn't even sleep last night. It was too hard being dishonest, after I learned so much at Daytop."

I'm not sure how that health-club manager responded when Suzie told him she wouldn't be coming back. He might have been angry. Or he might have had some secret admiration for this young woman who did the right thing.

That happens all the time when people on the outside come into contact with Daytop residents. Frequently, the people come away impressed. Some years ago, a New York City police officer stopped by to see me. He asked if I had a minute and said he wanted to tell me a story. He explained that the day before, he had been posted in Brooklyn, on Schermerhorn Street, on traffic patrol.

A Daytop van came along. A young man was driving and another young man was in the passenger seat. There was a stop sign at the corner where the officer was.

"I'm sure they didn't see it," he told me. "It was blocked by a UPS truck." In any event, the two Re-entry residents went through the corner without coming to a stop.

"I pulled them over," the officer said. "I asked for license and registration. I don't know what it was, but something about these kids piqued my interest. So I asked them what this word Daytop meant that was written on the side of the van, and they began to tell me about your program.

"They had such a wonderful sparkle to them, such honesty and a rare wholesomeness. Before I knew it, we had been talking for half an hour.

"I was so enthused, so impressed with them, it made me wish I had them for my own sons. So I told them, 'Don't worry about the ticket. I won't complete it. I'll just throw it away.'"

But the driver wouldn't hear of it. "Officer," he said, "please give us the ticket. We ran the stop sign. We made a mistake. In Daytop, we're bound to own up to our mistakes. When I get back to the house, the other people will give me a hard time about it. They might give me some extra work. They'll tell me I have to learn lessons from the mistakes of life. I must do that. That is part of my growth. So please give me the ticket."

The officer said he argued with the resident. But the young man was insistent. So he did what the kid wanted, and he handed the ticket to him.

"Then, I went home that night," the cop said. "I told my wife about it. And I was just so intrigued that I had to come here today."

He pulled a business-size envelope out of the pocket of his jacket.

"I want you to accept this from me for the work that you're doing," he said. In the envelope was a check for a hundred dollars from a New York City police officer whom we had never met before. But he had a brief contact with two of our Re-entry residents, who were missionaries, really, for this thing we call "Daytop living."

Encouragement and positive reinforcement of this sort make our job easier. They help fortify the residents when their new values are tested in truly difficult ways. But the contrast between the worlds inside and out can still be tough at times.

Here they are, getting readjusted to day-to-day life. Things are going nicely. With that open attitude, most of our kids don't have much trouble making friends. They work hard, and their employers love them. Some of these young people, don't forget, went many years without a whole lot of affection in their lives. Now, they are receiving praise and admiration all the time.

Then, they come back to the house at night—and the demanding side of the Daytop love reasserts itself. Sooner or later, every one of them is pulled up on some minor infraction. Maybe they didn't put their clothes away neatly, or they were brusque with another member of the family. At Daytop, don't forget, these things are treated like serious offenses.

It's a tricky combination, this merging of inside and out. By day, they are in the working world, where they are getting all this positive reinforcement and occasionally facing these real challenges. Then, every night they're back at Daytop, where we're still fine-tuning the product, pointing out how they can grow and what mistakes they've made.

But it works only if the people in Re-entry are relating honestly to each other about the things they are going through, especially the setbacks and the disappointments. Facing these things squarely is much more important than whatever actual mistake or infraction the resident might have made.

Unhappily, we've seen the results that are possible when people try to hold back in this turmoil. The story that comes first to my mind is about a young man named Cleveland and what happened to him in Re-entry B.

When the time comes for residents to start looking for work, we deliberately have them set up at least one interview with someone who doesn't know anything about drugs except for the silliness that's printed in the papers, someone who is sure to say, "Get lost, kid. Don't call us. We'll call you."

That way, Re-entry residents get to experience rejection. It helps teach them how to confront the disappointments that are an inevitable part of life.

Cleveland arranged an appointment to see a man who owned an electrical contracting business, a real SOB. The man's rotten temper was legendary. He had already rejected several of our residents, and we figured he was a safe bet. He never took a single kid from Daytop, and he gave all the applicants an incredibly hard time.

Well, he flipped over Cleveland. He loved the kid, just raved about him. And I remember, later, we said to this fellow, "Hey, listen, let him learn. Don't baby him." But he became like a father to Cleveland. He didn't want to hear it.

Cleveland had been working about eight months. One Friday night, we got a call from the boss. "Cleveland's not back with the truck," the man said. "I know he sometimes stops by Daytop because he loves the people there, and I want him to do that because he gets good energy from the kids."

"I'll check," I told him, and I called him back and said no one had seen Cleveland.

We called around to some of the other houses, and Cleveland hadn't been to any of them.

We finally found him at ten o'clock, his boss and I. The van was in Red Hook, in Brooklyn, and Cleveland was in the back. His heroin works were next to him on the floor of the van. He had died of an overdose.

We didn't know it, but Cleveland had just learned his father had died. His dad had suffered from serious diabetes and heart trouble. For seven weeks, he had been in a hospital intensive-care unit. Cleveland's mother died when he was twelve. His dad was the only relative he had. But the prospect of his father's dying so terrified Cleveland that he never allowed himself to think about it. Sadly, he never brought up the subject in his evening Re-entry group.

We thought Cleveland was ready to face life without drugs. He wasn't. And we learned all over again how fragile life is. It took me, personally, a very long time to recover from Cleveland's death.

Some of these young people are so lovable. But you cannot get too emotionally involved. You can't baby them. You must let them walk. You must let them run. And you must let them fall. It's a hard lesson for all of us. But you must let them fall.

Now, I would never blame his boss for Cleveland's death. Cleveland's demons were mostly inside. But the rest of us have to remember that being too gentle with these kids, too sweet with them, doesn't do anybody any good.

Thankfully, experiences like Cleveland's are more the exception than the rule. Being open in group—especially about the tough things—is the best safety valve we have. Over the years, we've learned some other lessons from our mistakes. And we've discovered ways to make Re-entry a more effective process.

One thing we have institutionalized is an intensive process for evaluating how well the residents are adjusting to Re-entry. This is especially important during Phase B, when those first "baby steps" out into the world are being taken. How are your social relationships? How well do you manage your finances? Have you learned to budget? Are you continuing to show responsibility toward the family? How are you getting along with members of the opposite sex? How does your employer feel about you? Are you being open and honest in group?

All these questions can sometimes strike the residents as nagging.

But we've discovered that the microscope has to stay in focus. Sometimes, the family will urge the resident to work harder in a certain area. Sometimes, the family will object to certain friends. Sometimes, the family will steer the resident toward or away from a certain job.

We've discovered, for instance, that self-employment is not usually a good idea for our people, especially at first. It is important for them to subject themselves to the discipline of working for someone else, for a company with rules that must be followed and standards that must be met.

For the same reason, big money from a job like construction also isn't so good. That sends the resident back to the old addict's way of thinking—immediate compensation, instant gratification, the magic that drugs were supposed to hold.

Some of the most growth-producing jobs are actually relatively menial positions, steady work for steady pay. Residents who want to be doctors or lawyers or computer designers, say, should place these goals fourth or fifth on their lists. "Your dream job doesn't have to be your first job," we tell the residents. "Engage in the discipline of working. Progress one step at a time."

Success at Daytop, of course, is never guaranteed. And this fact applies to Re-entry as much as it does to all the other stages of treatment.

Sometimes people fail. They aren't ready for the responsibility of heading back out into society. Sometimes they need to be re-cycled back Upstate for a few more months, before being brought back to try again.

This is terribly disappointing to a Re-entry resident, whose peers are all returning to the outside world. But sometimes people just need more work.

"Your life is a very important thing," we tell people in this position. "You come into the world all alone. You leave the world all alone. And your life is very important. So the family feels that you should go back Upstate for a little while so you can evaluate what's happened and figure out how you can better cope."

This is a loving recommendation. And in a few months, they'll come back, armed with those lessons, and do much better the second time. It's like buying insurance for the future.

The truth of the matter, though, is that for most addicts—even Daytop's biggest success stories—recovery is a process that never ends. They must continue to grow for the rest of their lives.

That's why the door at Daytop is always open.

I remember one day a few years ago, a fellow showed up with his wife and children. He was living then in Cincinnati. He had graduated from Daytop twelve or fourteen years before.

"We're having a crisis in our family," he said. "I'm not going to run away from it. Can I go up to Swan Lake with my family and confront this problem in Daytop groups?" He hardly knew anybody there anymore. Just a couple of staff people from his day were left. But that didn't matter, he told me.

"The energy of the place," he said. "Daytop always taught me to run to—not to run away from."

So he and his family spent a couple of days at Swan Lake.

They talked about his problem. He cut it up into little parts. And he dealt with each and every part.

He wrote a lovely letter later to the Daytop family when he got back to Ohio, thanking us for being there.

This graduate hadn't used drugs for many years. The problems he was facing had nothing to do with that. They had to do with family finances and the man's career.

But then, Daytop isn't about drugs, really. It's a school for living. It's a revolution in mental-health treatment. Its applications, I've always thought, go much wider than drug abuse. It creates the healing environment. It creates a support system. And over the years, that's how we've rebuilt those thousands of lives.

Often these successes look like miracles. Sometimes, though, they fly right off of the chart. I don't know how else to describe the story of Bruce.

I first heard his name in a telephone call that came unexpectedly one day from a probation officer in New Jersey. The P.O. explained that he was calling about a young man who was an inmate at Rahway, the state's toughest prison. The prisoner had done three years for a string of drug-related burglaries and before that had been a heroin addict for seven years.

His mother and father had been killed in a plane crash when Bruce was just eleven. An only child with no other family but an aged great-aunt, he had bounced from foster home to foster home and never quite fit in at any one of them.

Convinced that life had sold him short, Bruce began blocking out the pain with drugs. The burglaries brought excitement and helped finance the drugs.

"I don't think he belongs here," the probation officer told me when he called. "I think he belongs with you. If you're willing to take him at Daytop, he's yours. I can get the corrections department to go along."

We sent a team out to Rahway to interview Bruce. They saw some promise in him, a personal motivation, a commitment to change his life. They brought him back to my office.

I remember the expression on Bruce's face and the tears rolling down when he thanked me for getting him out of jail. He was just so pleased to be away from Rahway, he said, and he began telling me the story of his troubled childhood.

I cut him off quick.

"Bruce," I snapped, "who told you that your parents owed you anything? You could have the most wonderful parents. You could have the richest parents. Still, you could fall on your face. If you don't believe me, we can walk right out of this office, and I can introduce you to Daytop residents who came from highly respected families—and they still turned to drugs.

"Every generation has to take its own oars and row its boat alone. Stop feeling sorry for yourself, Bruce."

With tears rolling down his cheeks, Bruce intruded. "That's just what I have been doing all my life," he said.

Bruce loved Daytop, with its values and discipline.

He graduated in sixteen months, not the usual eighteen to twenty-two.

He won a scholarship to one of New Jersey's leading universities and graduated summa cum laude. In 1975, he applied for medical school, a year that the competition was especially tough. He was accepted at five schools and decided to go to the one with the most rigorous program, Columbia.

Today, he is an orthopedic surgeon at a big medical center in California.

And he adheres to Daytop's philosophy of total openness. He told the truth—the whole truth—about his past.

WHY IT WORKS 11

> *I believe it is by discovering and affirming the being in ourselves that some inner certainty will become possible. In contrast to the psychologies that conclude with theories about conditioning, mechanisms of behavior and instincted drives, I maintain that we must go below these theories and discover the person, the being to whom these things happen.*
>
> —Rollo May, *Discovery of Being*

Daytop's response to drug addiction is not something that was cooked up in the mind of a single, brilliant theorist. It has grown, organically, over the past thirty years.

Some elements of our concept were taken from Sigmund Freud and other insightful students of the human psyche. Some elements were borrowed from Synanon, Alcoholics Anonymous, and other treatment programs that arrived on the scene before we did. We are not shy about giving credit where credit is due.

A big part of what we know, however, we had to learn ourselves, day by day, in the real world of drug addiction, from the experiences of our residents and staff. Every one of those lessons was then time tested in the human laboratory we call Daytop Village.

At Daytop, we have always tried to avoid the temptation to over-intellectualize about what we do. What makes Daytop special is not the theoretical purity of our concept. What makes us special is that, most of the time, our concept works.

But there are some underlying questions. Unless we can come up with meaningful answers for them, we will never be able to spread the lessons of Daytop around the world or bring help to as many others as we possibly can.

What kinds of people are susceptible to addiction? How did they get that way? What has to happen before they can make fundamental changes in their lives? Why does our brand of treatment so often succeed? Conversely, why does it sometimes fail? These are all complicated questions. But thankfully, we've been mulling them over for a long time now, and we've been lucky enough to benefit from the guidance of some very keen minds.

People like Daniel Casriel have been there for us.

More than anyone else, Casriel helped ground our work in psychological theory. He helped us, in other words, to articulate in a conceptual way why it is we do what we do.

Casriel was the psychiatrist who stumbled into the Synanon house in Connecticut that same Saturday morning in 1959 that I did. He had studied drug addiction since the 1940s. He had been a consultant to various government programs and had treated hundreds of addicts in his private practice. Like everyone else back then, he was groping around for something that would work.

In his initial visits to Synanon, Casriel had seen some reason for hope. He was the first and—it turned out—the last professional investigator to be given a relatively free rein in studying Synanon's methods. He went on to write a book about the group's early achievements, *So Fair a House,* which was published in 1963. By the time the book came out, though, Casriel was already beginning to have his own misgivings about Synanon's increasingly authoritarian tone. This was just as Daytop was being rescued from its rocky first year of existence, and Casriel jumped at the chance to play a leading role. He became Daytop's first psychiatric director and remained a chief architect of our program until 1971. We suffered a severe loss in his untimely death in 1983.

Casriel came to the subject of drug addiction from the same perspective as most American psychiatrists. He had been greatly influenced by Freud's explanations of neurosis and psychosis, those two primary forms of mental illness. Casriel also believed strongly in the power of Freudian psychotherapy. Like many psychiatrists, he embraced the "adaptational" theory of human behavior: that, in general, people behave in ways they believe will enable them to achieve pleasure and avoid pain.

By the early 1960s, however, Casriel had grown discouraged with psychiatry's obvious failure to impact upon drug addiction. The psychiatrists weren't having any more luck than the physicians or the social workers or the penologists or any of the other "experts" who had been convinced they held the cure.

Something was obviously wrong with the addicts he was seeing. Casriel knew that. It was something that went far deeper than the mere decision to use drugs. But what was it?

Most addicts didn't exhibit the classic signs of psychosis or neurosis that Freud had warned about. They didn't even tend to complain all that much, except when they were having trouble finding drugs. And after many hours on the analyst's couch, rarely did the addicts seem to get well.

But Casriel's eyes had been opened at Synanon, and he saw the same hopeful signs at Daytop. None of this had been predicted in the psychiatric literature. But here were hardened drug addicts, living in highly structured communities, who were learning to rid their lives of drugs.

"The number-one factor in the understanding of drug addiction," Casriel wrote in the Synanon book, "is the realization that drug abuse is not in itself a disease but merely a manifestation of underlying psychologic or emotional" problems. Addiction is not, in other words, something that all of us are equally susceptible to as we go about our daily lives.

Addicts, he concluded, suffer from a special "character disorder" that is different from the varieties of mental illness that Freud laid out. The addicts' basic problem is immaturity. "Addicts," Casriel wrote, "are emotional infants"—locked in adult bodies. Whatever their chronological age, most of them are fundamentally unable to cope with the day-to-day stresses of the adult world.

To someone who suffers from this kind of emotional immaturity, any demand or challenge or difficulty in life presents itself as a monumental threat. What an emotionally mature person might experience as slight irritation the emotional child sees as a terrible menace. Such people will try to eliminate stress at almost any cost.

Usually, they will call upon one of three remedies for stress.

Some people get angry, and that anger often explodes into violence. A classic case was that man down in Atlanta who had been out of work for several months. The telephone company kept sending bills to his house, and this made him upset. So he climbed into his automobile and drove it through the plate-glass window of the local phone-company office. That was his way of dealing with stress.

Other emotionally immature people are so scared by stress that they literally run away. They disappear. They flee from their families and their bills. They keep moving. For some reason, such people seem to congregate at the extremities of the nation—down to Florida, say, or out in California. Sometimes, they leave the country altogether. That is their way of avoiding the pressures of adult life.

But there is a third way that emotionally immature people react to stress, and this is the one favored by most drug addicts and alcoholics. This is the one that Freud overlooked. They withdraw. They react like the turtle pulling its head into its shell. They use chemicals to shield themselves, to anesthetize their senses, to neutralize all the stress. They don't run from the world in the literal sense. They simply block it out.

For them, this eases the pain.

In our society, drugs and alcohol are the most readily available methods of emotional anesthesia. But if those substances weren't on hand, these people would no doubt find some substitute. To them, the stress of everyday living is just too great a burden to bear alone. They need that protective shell, that invisible psychic capsule they can hide inside.

Why would someone choose to withdraw like that?

Life, after all, inevitably includes some stress, and most people are not devastated by it. We all live with pressure and disappointment. Demands are always being made on us. The rent, or the house note, is due every month. The boss expects us to appear at work on time. Our spouses or our parents or our children are full of expectations. Why do these things hit some people so hard?

Like so much else in the realm of human psychology, this goes back to the individual's upbringing. Something important was missing on the road to maturity.

Think back to infancy. Almost all aspects of the infant's life were guided and controlled by the parents. The infant was expected to take almost no responsibility for his or her own care. Feeding, changing, emotional comfort—all of it was provided by the parents.

But as the child grew older, that parental control should have yielded to increasing self-control. The process is called maturation, and it works like this: One step at a time, the child faces bigger and bigger challenges. She learns to tie her shoes. He learns to make his bed. They learn to exercise increasing degrees of responsibility in all corners of their lives. And so by the age of seventeen or eighteen or nineteen, most children can handle most of the basics of life.

In some families, however, children are deprived of challenges. Generally, this doesn't stop them from learning to talk or eat or go to the bathroom. But when it comes to the far more difficult process of building emotional maturity, these children fall far short. They never learned to live up to expectations. They never learned to deal with demands. They were never challenged adequately. So they never grew.

The problem wasn't the parents' motives. In most cases, they were doing what they thought was best. Unfortunately, they had a misguided sense of what love means. They remembered the hard things about their own upbringings, all the luxuries they were denied. They wanted their children to have an easier time. So the parents didn't demand. They merely gave. They didn't tell the child, "Make your bed." They said, "I'll make it for you." Instead of insisting that the teenage son or daughter work in a fast-food restaurant to earn money for a new car, the parent said, "Happy high-school graduation. Here are the keys."

It's a seductive process. Frequently, parents don't even notice it happening. Cutting off this outpouring of unearned generosity, they tell themselves, would demonstrate some lack of love. "Besides," the parents will say, "the neighbors are giving their children de-signer outfits and two-hundred-dollar sneakers. Why should my kids be deprived?" The parents usually have the finest of intentions. They genuinely believe they are helping their kids. But the love they are giving makes no demands. It is a consuming, destructive love. They don't realize the deep damage it does.

What they end up with is a nineteen-year-old son or daughter who has an emotional age of eight. And no eight-year-old can pos-sibly handle the stress of being an adult.

This process, Casriel wrote, produces young people who are "too impotent to run to avoid the pain or danger and too defenseless and vulnerable to fight to remove it." Instead, they follow that third strategy for eliminating stress: they "withdraw by use of drugs into the very unreal world of imagined safety."

That chemical capsule is a comfortable one. It is warm. It is relatively secure. It keeps the pain of everyday living at bay. This is one of the reasons drug addicts seldom have the internal moti-vation to turn themselves around. They may see their lives in tur-moil; but where's the motivation when their senses have been so dulled by drugs?

This has its attractions, of course. But that protective capsule has some unintended side effects, as well. For one thing, it chokes off the individual's growth.

"A human personality, like a flower, cannot grow in a closed box," Casriel wrote when he came back to the topic in 1971. "When an individual utilizes withdrawal early in life, or even in later life, uses emotional detachment as a total defense mechanism, his char-acter stops growing, regresses and atrophies."

But "realistically, he is quite isolated, incapacitated and imprisoned. His original fortress has become his stockade. The longer the individual stays in his own jail, the thicker the walls become through secondary encapsulation, with the result that the individual becomes less and less able to cope with the problems of everyday living."

For such people, Casriel concluded, "the standard psychoanalytic techniques using introspection and observation are useless. The individual patient, though he hears, cannot be reached. Though he knows, he will not change. He will avoid the truth with or without outright lies."

A different kind of treatment is called for. It must be something more intense, something far-reaching, something that can crack through that drug-hardened shell.

That's what the "therapeutic community" of Daytop is designed to do.

This term, therapeutic community, is heard often at Daytop. At its most basic, it means a group of people who have come together for the purpose of self-discovery and self-improvement. They make up what might be thought of as a healing family, walking through the rugged but extremely caring and supportive terrain of humanizing, challenging self-help.

The roots of the therapeutic community go far back into history. The clans of ancient peoples operated in some ways as therapeutic communities, even if the concept was never articulated like that. The great O. Hobart Mowrer has written brilliantly on the striking manner in which the early church was organized, much like what we now think of as modern therapeutic communities. I was fortunate enough to do my graduate field work on AA under Mowrer's supervision at the University of Illinois.

"Early Christianity was basically a *small-group movement* in which alienated, sinful, 'neurotic' persons confessed before and did penance under the guidance of the particular 'congregation' (or 'house church') to which they belonged or wished to belong." The caring group, then, moved to support changes or improvements in behavior. "From all indications, this type of experience was highly 'therapeutic,' and it seems likely that this early version of Christianity survived and spread . . . because it was redemptive and rehabilitative in an intensely practical, psychologically and socially important way."

Imagine how much more vital the church would be today if it hadn't loosened this powerful grip on believers.

But the early church didn't last. In 325, Constantine the Great, fearing the disintegration of the Roman Empire, called the Council of Nicea and offered the Christian leaders a deal they could hardly refuse: He would put an end to three centuries of persecution—indeed, he would make Christianity the official religion of the state—if the churchmen would give him a single, monolithic statement of their faith, with all the controversy and dissension ironed out.

Mowrer describes the predictable result. "Christianity now became obligated to strive for massive popular, 'universal' (which is what 'catholic' means) appeal and as a result, it began to lose its pristine redemptive efficacy," he writes. Among the first and biggest losses was public confession. "Because quasi-public confession (before a small group or 'congregation') was humiliating and painful, it was gradually abandoned in favor of private 'auricular' confession (to a priest only), and psychologically and socially adequate penance for personal sin and guilt was also conveniently replaced."

What the faithful got instead were the recitation of simple prayers, opportunities to do quiet works of charity and, perhaps, the chance to purchase indulgences, as Martin Luther contended. But then, Protestantism went even further to isolate the sinner seeking forgiveness and reconciliation. It took away the confessor and made quiet, solitary admission of guilt in one's own private place the substitute for the original healing group church.

This process of transition took several centuries. But the church has never fully recaptured this therapeutic power it lost. Only in comparatively recent times has the idea been picked up again. And this time it wasn't by theologians at all.

The idea that a community could in itself be a useful therapeutic tool began gaining some currency in the mental-health field. True, we've had psychiatric hospitals for generations, but only recently has anyone thought of the mental hospital as more than just a place to lodge patients while they are treated.

In the late 1940s, the British psychiatrist Maxwell Jones was experimenting with what he called "humanizing institutional treatment settings" at Dingleton Hospital in Scotland and Henderson Hospital in London. He found that, in important ways, the patients could help cure each other. Synanon learned that lesson and expanded on it. So did Daytop.

The therapeutic communities that Daytop has created at its Upstate houses are designed to teach the residents a healthier, more natural way of confronting stress. We do it by closing off the three unhealthy options and insisting that the residents travel through the family process a second time. This time, it is the Daytop family, where demanding love and earned achievement prevail. The prime target is emotional maturity.

By so doing, the residents ultimately learn to re-create themselves.

All violence (arising from the emotion of anger) is absolutely prohibited, even the threat of violence. That takes care of unhealthy option number one.

As for option number two—flight (arising from the emotion of fear)—we don't prohibit it outright. Daytop, after all, is not a prison, and residents are not locked inside. But we make the cost of fleeing so unattractively high that most people choose to stay. "That's the route you followed on the street," we tell the residents. "You had all the freedom in the world, and you couldn't handle it. You constantly ran away. If you want to keep doing that, you don't belong at Daytop. But think long and hard before you go. We'll make it very difficult for you to get back in. And even if you do return, you'll have to prove yourself ten times over to achieve the place you have today." Some people do leave, of course. But for most residents, this becomes an unattractive option.

And the third unhealthy option for dealing with stress—withdrawal—falls under Daytop's other cardinal rule. No chemicals are permitted at Daytop anywhere, any time. No drugs, no alcohol. We are also strict about a lesser, nonchemical form of withdrawal. Daytop residents, for instance, are not permitted to just sit around their bedrooms alone. And if one person is sitting at a table in the dining room, other residents are expected to join him or her.

So, in effect, Daytop doesn't leave its residents with much choice. They are pressured to work all the way up from the bottom of this rigid family structure Daytop has created, a family where the love is most assuredly of the challenging kind. And the new residents are the babies of the house, encouraged to live under a strict set of parentally imposed controls. Their "new parents" are the staff and older members.

"Why?"—the new residents always want to know when they learn about some new oppressive-sounding rule.

"Because you are a baby," they are told.

In fact, they are treated exactly like babies whose parents won't let them run too close to the street or play with matches. They might hurt themselves. "Who would jam a dirty needle into a vein in an arm?" they are asked. "Who would swallow pills that could easily be lethal? Who would suck on a crack pipe that contained a mind-freezing poison? Who would do such stupid things?"

The answer has to be harsh.

"A baby. Nobody but a baby. No one else would be that dumb. You don't have a drug problem. You have a baby problem. Now, you're here to learn."

Just about every element of the Daytop treatment program—from Morning Meeting until the last encounter group at night—is designed to teach the lessons of emotional maturity.

The residents must learn to deal with stress as mature people do. They learn to plan their lives with an eye to the future. They learn to express their feelings. They learn to manage their differences with others by talking things out. They learn to channel their frustrations in directions that are productive.

The daily "pull ups" are only one example of this process. At Daytop, if a resident has a disagreement with someone else in the house, we have a structured system for dealing with that: write that person's name next to yours on a slip of paper and put the paper in the encounter box. The two of you can hash out your differences in the next encounter group.

This, obviously, isn't precisely the way people on the outside deal with their differences. But it teaches important lessons to addicts who didn't learn them the first time around. It teaches the residents how to delay gratification, how to control emotions, how to deal with things in an appropriate forum, how to express what is on their minds.

It teaches, in other words, maturity in confronting the day-to-day stresses of life.

This strict system of "parental control" lasts through the first four or five months Upstate. Then, slowly, it is eased. And the gradual transference to a more mature level of self-control, which failed to take hold in the addict's original family, is given a second chance.

By the time ten or twelve months have gone by, the residents find themselves learning to organize their own lives and taking responsibility for others. Then, they'll be ready for the "stress house" of Re-entry, to test how well the process has taken hold.

"The addict has to be taught, step-by-step, how to live in the world of the adult," Casriel wrote. "He has to be given the opportunity and the training to develop a mature personality."

There is so much that needs to be done. Daytop has to teach the addict how to "grow up and develop emotionally, socially, culturally, ethically, morally, sexually and vocationally. This is no small undertaking, but nothing less will suffice."

It is dangerous to generalize about the kinds of people who come to Daytop. Demographically speaking, we get all types.

We get rich people and poor people and lots of people in between. They are Catholic and Protestant and Jewish and Muslim and almost anything else there is. Daytop is run by a priest, but it is a nonsectarian organization. Some of our residents are highly educated; some can barely read. They arrive from the city and the country and the suburb. Their heritage is a rainbow coalition of ethnic and racial groups. They are gay and straight. They are at almost every imaginable stage of life—anywhere from their early teens to their forties or fifties or beyond.

As for the kinds of drugs they used, our people come in having taken every drug there is—often many of them at the same time. Heroin, cocaine, crack, hallucinogens, prescription medications, alcohol—you name it, they've shot, snorted, smoked, eaten or drunk it. And the treatment they receive at Daytop isn't much affected by the kind of drugs they were using when they came in the door. No doubt, next month or next year some new chemical will come along.

Daytop doesn't target the drug. What we do is aimed at the person hiding behind the drug. And the principles apply regardless of the addict's particular substance of choice.

Our research department gathers statistics on our population. On any given day, there are approximately 2,400 people in the program. In addition, about 1,600 family members are receiving counseling sessions with Daytop staff.

On average, 327 people are admitted to the program each month, about 40 percent of them to residential treatment. The rest come to Daytop for an array of outpatient services.

Here's the current breakdown: 72 percent are male, 28 percent female. (The proportion of women has been growing a little every year.) The average age is twenty-nine. At any given time, we have more than a thousand people on the waiting list. Of those who call, half will go to the outpatient services we call "Daytop Outreach." The median wait for a bed is forty days.

These numbers illustrate just how big and diverse the Daytop family has become. But, please, don't be fooled by all that diversity. There is something that the majority of our people share—besides a crippling problem with drugs. Almost all of them come from families that failed.

Some of these failed families are a kind of popular stereotype. They are poor and headed by a single parent, inevitably the mother. She has inadequate education, as do the children, and few marketable skills. The neighborhood is rough. Housing is substandard. Money is tight, except for the occasional windfalls from the commerce of drugs. Racism may well be an additional burden, and rarely is a positive male role model anywhere on the scene. Mother is so busy looking after the barest essentials, the children grow up without the discipline and guidance that they need. Even if mom has the love and the energy and the desire to be a successful parent, chances are she lacks many of the most basic techniques and the time it takes to parent well.

The hopelessness and pathology of this kind of upbringing has been written about for generations now. And its burdens are real, indeed. When speaking about young people raised in such an environment, you really can't talk about *re*habilitation. Habilitation would be a better word. They have to learn many of the basic skills of living for the very first time.

Before Daytop can do anything else for such youngsters, we must supply the love and attention and guidance and discipline that was absent at home. And we do that.

But there is a second kind of failed family we see just as often at Daytop, although these failures can sometimes be harder to detect at first. Rehabilitation is sometimes a possibility in such families, but the problems can still run just as deep.

These are middle-class families, or even upper class. To outsiders, these families might appear trouble free. The children have all the social opportunities; education and other cultural advantages are available; the housing and the neighborhoods are decent; and the other middle-class trappings are there for them.

Something is missing nonetheless. Like their counterparts in the ghetto, these children also lack adequate discipline.

The reason isn't an absence of love. These youngsters get plenty of love. But they get the wrong kind of love. They get a consuming, destructive love, a love that says, "Give Johnny the things I didn't have when I grew up. Give Johnny anything he wants."

The problem is a misapplied love, a malintentioned love. What this produces is a parent who ends up acting more like a child than the child does. The resulting chaos has taken over Johnny's life.

Daytop begins to reverse that. Daytop begins immediately to teach a demanding love, a tough love, a love that says, "I love you so much that I want you to grow and become responsible." It's not a sympathetic love. It's a challenging love, and it's a very beautiful thing.

The power of this misapplied love may be one explanation for an odd fact we have noticed over the years about the young people who seek treatment at Daytop.

Most of them are either the firstborn or lastborn in their families. The firstborn is the little treasure that has arrived magically in the parents' lives—and nothing is ever going to hurt little Marilyn. The last child is the parents' lifelong ticket to youthfulness. So the baby cannot be permitted to ever grow up.

Those attitudes frequently get carried all the way through a child's upbringing, as the parents try to demonstrate their special love with overprotectiveness. The little darling is never allowed to mature.

One day soon after Daytop Village had opened, that towering psychologist Abraham Maslow came for a visit with two of his colleagues from Brandeis University. He asked many questions and stayed for most of the day. Later, in his final book, *The Further Reaches of Human Nature*, Maslow described Daytop as a beautiful place that had lessons for everyone—not just drug addicts.

"The process here basically poses the question of what people need universally," he wrote. "It seems to me that there is a fair amount of evidence that the things that people need as basic human beings are few in number. It is not very complicated. They need a feeling of protection and safety, to be taken care of when they are so young so that they feel safe. Second, they need a feeling of belongingness, some kind of family, clan or group, or something that they feel that they are in or belong to by right. Third, they have to have the feeling that people have affection for them, that they are worth being loved. And fourth, they must experience respect and esteem. And that's about it. . . . Could it be that Daytop is effective because it provides an environment where these feelings are possible? . . . Isn't it a pity we're not all addicts; because if we were, we could come to this wonderful place!"

Maslow and countless other visitors over the years have seen what a real jewel the therapeutic community can be, a utopian society where each member has accepted the responsibility for his life and for his brothers' and sisters' lives as well. The therapeutic community is a place without sympathy or attachments that are condescending or destructive.

It is a place where people are challenging themselves and each other to climb that hill together.

"Only you can do it," the residents are constantly reminded, "but you cannot do it alone."

KEEPING SCORE **12**

If a man does away with his traditional way of living and throws away his good customs, he had better first make certain that he has something of value to replace them.
(Old Basuto proverb, which appears in the lore of many African tribes of Bantu origin.)

—**Robert Ruark,** *Something of Value*

We get visitors all the time at Daytop. Psychiatrists show up. So do social workers and politicians and police officials and government bureaucrats and all sorts of other people.

We're happy to have them. These visits give people a chance to learn firsthand about the work we do and to meet our residents and staff. If our guests have time to visit one of the Daytop Outreach Centers or even one of the houses Upstate, we try to arrange that.

At some point during these visits, usually near the end, there's one question that almost always comes up.

"Well, this whole thing seems really beautiful," the person will say. "But what's your score? What's your success rate? How many people get through Daytop? How many of them leave Daytop cured?"

We Americans are like that, I suppose—focused on results, respectful of hard data, insistent on statistical support.

In a sense, the questions are a little unfair. Social workers are rarely asked, "How frequently do you succeed in reversing the ravages of poverty?" I don't think I've ever heard anyone ask a psychiatrist, "What percentage of your schizophrenic patients are cured at all, much less in eighteen months?" This is lucky for social workers and psychiatrists. In neither case would the numbers be very high. One percent, 2 percent. If the "success rates" of these conventional healing professions got that high, people would be calling them miracle workers. When it comes, say, to prison, I don't think anyone even holds out hope anymore that the penologists rehabilitate anyone.

But we get the question all the time. Perhaps it's because our approach is beyond the boundaries of these traditional turfs. Thankfully, we can be proud of our achievements, and we are pleased to answer these questions.

People deserve answers—the people who are thinking about coming into treatment and their families, as well as the government agencies, foundations, and individuals we call upon for financial support.

We have not forgotten the lessons of Synanon. We are open to outside scrutiny and outside verification of our claims. So here's how we go about measuring success—and how people who've been through Daytop stack up.

The concept of "success" in a drug-treatment program can be defined in any number of ways. We have come up with a demanding, triple scale. First and foremost, success at Daytop means living a drug-free life. Cutting back isn't enough. Just using occasionally isn't the point. The goal of Daytop is drug-free living. Before we'll call you a success, we want you completely off of drugs.

The second standard we use is "freedom from crime." No arrests, no convictions, no further involvement in the criminal activities that most drug addicts were drawn into.

The third part of the test is most subjective. It's what we call "positive life-style." Is the person living a productive life? Going to school? Holding a job? Maintaining healthy relationships with family and friends?

Those three ingredients go into the texture of what we call "success."

Even by this tough standard, our people score exceedingly well.

Our results aren't perfect. Some people don't get better. But of those who travel through Daytop to the finish, 88 percent meet all three prongs of the test. They are off drugs; they are out of crime; and they are living positive, productive lives.

Eighty-eight percent.

It's amazing when you think about it.

Eighty-eight percent of these hardened drug addicts living useful, socially productive lives. When they came to us, these were some of the toughest cases around. These were people who defied every previous attempt at treatment, who swatted off every single helping hand.

This 88 percent refers to our graduates, to the ones who see Daytop through. They completed Upstate treatment and stayed around through the three phases of Re-entry. The whole thing might have taken eighteen months or even a little more. These are the ones who got the full effect of what we have. And their rates of success are, of course, the best.

But as we've studied our numbers, another interesting fact has come to light: Even those who don't complete the program show significant benefits from the time they spent with us.

About half of the people who start treatment drop out at some time before graduation. There are all kinds of reasons for this. Some people feel they have already gotten the benefits from treatment and are ready to go off on their own. Others find a weak front among relatives or friends and return to their old drug habits. Still others leave because of a romance or some incident that took place in the house. In the heat of the moment, they are not thinking clearly and leave impetuously. (Of those who leave early, about 15 percent come back to us and another 5 percent go to one of our sister programs.)

But we have discovered that even these people derive some real benefits from Daytop treatment. The longer they stay, not surprisingly, the greater those benefits are.

Johns Hopkins did a research project a few years ago, looking at six Daytop-like therapeutic communities across the country. The study verified what our internal research department had found:

that 68 percent of the residents who stay for six months "succeed" according to our triple scale.

Those who stay for twelve months do markedly better—86 percent. This is almost—though not quite—as good as the performance of those who stay for graduation.

Just how far a little Daytop can go was driven home to me back in 1970. I had flown to Chicago to visit Dr. Edward Senay, one of the real heroes in drug treatment. Senay had fielded one of the nation's best urban drug programs, with an array of treatment designs and sample intakes.

I was picked up at O'Hare Airport by a young man who seemed very eager to speak with me.

"How do you know me?" I asked him after we'd both gotten into the car. "Were you ever in New York?"

"As a matter of fact, I was," he said. He explained he had grown up in Chicago and had begun using drugs early in his teens. "I was involved in a lot of crime in Chicago, and I took off one time. There was a lot of heat on me from the police and from some dealers I owed some money to. Anyway, I moved out of Chicago and went out to New York. While I was out there, I got into Daytop. I didn't stay. I was there for only twenty-four hours, and then I split. I wasn't ready, I guess you'd have to say."

But Daytop still made an important mark.

"In those twenty-four hours at Daytop, I saw for the first time some kind of light at the end of the tunnel I was in. Back before that, when I was using drugs, all I ever saw was a dark wall in front of me. I used to say the only time I was going to get through that wall was when I died."

But in twenty-four hours, Daytop had planted a possibility in this young man's mind. "I got into this program in Chicago because I knew that it could work," he said. "I had seen that at Daytop. I didn't do it then. I did not let it happen. Maybe I wasn't ready. I don't know. But I knew about the concept. I knew that this was a program that wasn't absorbed with the drug of use, but with the person and the problems compelling the person to use the drugs."

Interesting story, isn't it? We must not underestimate the value of exposure to Daytop. Twenty-four hours could do that. Six months or twelve months can do something even more extraordinary—even for those who never graduate.

We strongly encourage every resident to stick around for graduation. The longer the better—that rule still applies. But thankfully, Daytop is not an all-or-nothing affair.

The same thing, incidentally, has proven true at the ten Daytop Outreach Centers that we have established in the New York metropolitan area. Each center serves 150 or so young people. They receive day-care or night-care treatment similar to the residential regime, but tailored mostly to less-troubled adolescents. The success statistics parallel the scores on the residential side.

So how much does all this cost?

Very little, compared to the damage a drug addict wreaks on the people who love him and the people he lives around. And very little, compared to the various other alternatives that society has tried.

It costs $19,000 a year to keep someone in residence at Daytop. This includes just about everything: housing, food, clothing, transportation, medical care—and all aspects of treatment. Outpatient care comes to just $3,700.

Several factors help Daytop keep its costs low.

For one thing, the residents themselves cut the grass, shovel the snow, answer the phones, wash the dishes, and perform the thousands of other tasks that someone otherwise would have to be hired to do. At Daytop, these things are all part of treatment—steps on the responsibility ladder.

Second, the people we do hire are by and large with us out of commitment, not for high salaries. The program is run with relatively few high-priced professionals. A staff of psychiatrists and psychologists and physicians provides the technical, specialized services. But most of the day-to-day work is done by very skilled ex-addicts, who are paid much less. Many are themselves graduates of the program, people whose lives mirror the success of Daytop. To them, Daytop is not just a job. It's a calling. It's a way of paying back.

By comparison, keeping a teenager at the Spofford Youth Correctional Center, New York's largest juvenile prison, costs the state $56,000 a year. For that price, the young person is terrorized and abused in all sorts of unspeakable ways—and almost never rehabilitated. To keep an adult in state prison—say, at Attica—is also no bargain, about $35,000 a year.

The public mental hospitals are even more costly. New York State spends, on average, $68,000 a year to warehouse someone in one of these hellholes. Private mental hospitals are even pricier. Two hundred thousand dollars a year is not an uncommon fee.

I'm not saying the doors to America's psych wards and cell blocks should be swung open tomorrow. I'm not saying that all the patients and inmates should be marched off promptly to Daytop. Obviously, some people belong in prison or in a mental hospital.

But when you compare their success rates to Daytop's—or their price tags to ours—it's hard not to believe the balance should be tipped a little more in our direction.

One of the truly depressing facts of today's world is how programs like Daytop have to scratch for every nickel of public support, while the politicians clamor constantly for more and more Spoffords, more and more Atticas, more and more places to lock people up and throw away the key.

PULLING THE FAMILY IN 13

> ... *that, if a family has a chemical abuse problem, then its hierarchical arrangement is confused, the 'fit' between drug abuse and the family's pattern of interacting must be reduced to insure that relapse is less likely.*
>
> —Jay Haley, Problem-Solving Therapy, 9th World Conference of Therapeutic Communities, San Francisco, California, 1985

By the time Roger Watson was forty, he seemed to have everything a man could want.

He had three daughters and a son. He had enough money and material possessions to support his family through several generations of luxury. And he had the knowledge that all this worldly success was the fruit of his own intelligence and hard work.

Roger and I had been friends as children. He had grown up in a poor family in the Bronx, the sixth of seven children. His parents struggled to send him to parochial school, and that is where the two of us met. After high school, he did what many ambitious children from poor families do, when their parents don't have the money for college. He enlisted in the army.

He served all over the world—in Europe and Asia and the South Pacific and on the West Coast of the United States. His final tour was in the Bavarian Alps, just this side of the Austrian border.

Roger liked Europe. And when he finally put in his retirement papers, he decided to stay there for a while. The European economy was booming then, and Roger always had a good head for business. So he tried his hand at real estate development and then the wholesale-distribution business.

At one point, he maintained eighteen residences around the world, including his home base on an island off the coast of Spain.

He had a gigantic yacht in the Mediterranean and a steady flow of famous visitors.

One day, after some business meetings in Europe, I went to see my old friend. By this time, the three girls were into the teen years and his son had just turned ten.

I remember sitting at poolside, trying to talk, as this bratty kid was running around, screaming and demanding instant service from the household staff. "Spoiled" barely begins to describe what little Thomas was like.

"Your crown prince here is going to be in trouble," I said to the father at one point.

"Do you think so?" he asked.

"I know so," I told him.

Well, before I left, the ten-year-old boy had driven his father's Maserati into the swimming pool.

As the years went by, things only got worse. At fifteen, young Thomas got a driver's license and his own Corvette—with the father's help, of course. He was a terror on the road. Shortly after that, the father arranged for him to get a helicopter license, too. He used to get great pleasure buzzing the beaches of the island and making the tourists think he was about to crash.

Let me tell you, the kid did not want for much.

By this point, his three sisters had married and moved away. When Thomas went to visit them on holidays, he never took a commercial flight. He hired a private plane and had a chauffeured car waiting for him when he arrived.

It was probably nine or ten years after our poolside visit that the father called me out of the blue one day. He sounded terribly distraught. The reason, he said, was his son.

"I guess you were right," Roger said. "The boy has become a real problem." The father had just brought the young man to a famous psychiatric clinic in Cleveland because the boy was seriously into drugs. The admitting psychiatrist, who happened to be from Spain, interviewed both the father and the son.

"What's the problem?" he asked the father. And the father told him the boy is using drugs and spending, roughly, $46,000 a month on the drugs and other diversions.

The psychiatrist asked who pays the $46,000, and the father said, "I do."

The psychiatrist told the father that he was the one who really needed the help—not the son. And the father, outraged at what the doctor said, stormed out of the hospital in a huff. A week later, he called me.

"The boy really needs help," he said. "Maybe I do too. I don't know. I brought the boy to London. He's in a clinic there now, where they just keep him heavily sedated on Valium all day. I think Daytop would probably be a better idea."

I told the father that I would be pleased to take his son, but only under two conditions: First, that he cut off all the boy's money completely, and second, that from now on I would be the boy's father. He would begin taking orders from me.

The father agreed immediately and arranged for the flight to New York. Thirty pieces of Louis Vuitton luggage arrived in my office on a Friday afternoon, along with precious young Thomas.

He was so stoned when he arrived, I knew that we wouldn't be able to pierce the fog of sedation right away. So I arranged for him to stay with friends over the weekend. He promised he would not take any more drugs and he would show up at my office again on Monday morning at exactly eight.

Well, he decided to spend the weekend on a cocaine-and-vodka binge with a few New York celebrities he had met at his father's house in Spain—including the actress-daughter of a famous writer and the wife of a high government official from Canada.

He didn't show up at my office for the Monday morning appointment, and I didn't hear from him at all that day. At two o'clock the next morning, an urgent call came into the parish house. Thomas was on the line. He explained that he was over at the Hotel Carlyle, and he didn't have any money for the bill.

"We're not going to pay," I told him, although this didn't seem to cause much alarm. "I'm your father now, remember?"

"It's all right," he said. "I just slit my wrists anyway. When can you get down here?"

"No," I told him. "I'm not coming at all. You want to cut your wrists, you can cut your wrists." Then, I called the manager at the Carlyle, and I asked him to check the suite of young Thomas Watson.

The boy had done some cutting all right, but they were just superficial cuts. The hotel manager called back and said he had sent Thomas over to Lenox Hill Hospital, to have his cuts sewn up.

I went over to the hospital the following morning, smiled at him, and said: "Come with me. This has gone on about long enough. You're going to Daytop now." I got him a seat on a van that was going up to the Millbrook house. And that was the last I saw of young Thomas for six weeks or so.

It was not, I am told, an easy transition. Here was one of the wealthiest young men in the world, confronted for the first time in his life by strangers, kids from every level of American life. They were demanding to know where his life was going. They treated him with no special respect, just the usual conditional love that is part of Daytop life. They demanded that he start growing up.

He was taken aback at the beginning, but he slowly began to blend into the family.

The next time I was up at Millbrook, I heard this lovely British-accented voice calling me. It was Thomas, of course. "May I speak with you?" he asked politely.

"You'd better ask your director," I told him. The director said he could speak to me for four minutes. So we walked around the grounds and had a brief conversation.

The Europeans overwork the word "incredible." But that was the word he chose. "This is incredible," he said. "This is really incredible. The love is really incredible. But I don't really belong here."

So I looked at him and said, "You know, your father was a poor boy from the Bronx. He busted his rear end to make something of himself, went into the army, went through basic training, served in the military and became very successful. Why do you think you're an exception? Why don't you start learning about life. You have to begin to pull your own weight, climb your own hills, fashion your own life."

And I looked at my watch and the four minutes were up. I said, "Go back in the house." And he went back in.

There was a tremendous culture shock there of learning what life was all about. Now, he had no escape hatch. He was being confronted on all sides by kids who really cared for him, and that's the beautiful thing about coming into Daytop.

In our society—in most societies, in fact—parents are expected to accomplish an extraordinary combination of things. They have to be part clergyman, part maid, part doctor, part nurse, part psychiatrist, part teacher and part referee.

Oh yes, and part taxi driver, too.

Unfortunately, the new baby doesn't arrive with an instruction manual for mom and dad. We just cross our fingers and expect the art of parenting to be learned almost by osmosis.

Compare that with how our society goes about preparing people for the other helping professions—law, medicine, social work, and so on.

Typically, professional training starts with many years of formal education, usually including college and graduate school. That is often followed by some kind of internship or apprentice program, during which the neophyte's skills are honed under the guidance of an experienced practitioner.

Only then are these newly minted professionals let loose on the world.

Yet when it comes to training parents, we throw up our hands and hope for the best.

Maybe the new mother will pick up a few tricks from her mother. Or maybe not. Maybe the new father will read a book or two about being a parent. Or again, maybe not.

All of it is left largely to chance. Government funding? Almost none is available for parent training. Every state in the nation has a state-supported law school. How many have graduate programs in parenthood?

Given all that is stacked against them, some parents do miraculously well. Most leave a lot to be desired, however. They were never even given the basic tools required for success.

One of our parents wrote a magnificent story about her drug-addicted adolescent son, who went through the Daytop house at Millbrook.

In painful detail, she described how she had babied the boy all through his growing-up years. She remembered one particular day, when he was just ten and his goldfish had died.

The mother noticed this right after she got up that morning, while her son was brushing his teeth.

But she couldn't bear the thought of her young son facing the awful trauma of death. So she didn't say a word. She just pulled a cover over the fish bowl and hustled the boy out of the house.

While he was at school that day, she rushed from one pet shop to another until she found a fish that almost perfectly matched the one that had died. She paid for it and carried it back to the house.

By the time her son got home from school that afternoon, the new fish was swimming happily where the old had.

Her son never knew the difference.

An act of love, right?

In a sense, it certainly was.

But what a terrible thing to do to a child! What a tragedy to squander an opportunity like that!

The mother had deprived her son of an important maturing experience. Death happens in life. The only way we learn to deal with it is to begin in small and simple ways.

Instead, the mother had engaged in exactly the same pathological fashion Daniel Casriel had written about.

Remember what he said? Maturation is the transference from *parental-imposed controls*—"do your homework, clean your room, wash the dishes, mow the lawn"—to *self-imposed controls*. Ultimately, children have to become the captains of their own ships. They have to make their own decisions and become, to use a phrase from politics, self-governing entities.

Unfortunately, this process takes place in the stormiest part of a young person's life, during adolescence. And unfortunately, parents more often than not look at their children with the eyes of protecting them from any hardship—in particular, the hardships that the parents themselves experienced in their lives. This is only natural. The parent loves the child. Most parents want only the best for their children.

But this wonderful instinct blinds many parents to the real goal of parenting—not softening a child's journey through life but giving the child the wings to fly alone.

Most of the time, the parents are acting out of what they believe is love. But it is not healthy love. In Daytop, we call it consuming-destructive love. Rather than going through the hassle of getting the daughter to clean up her bedroom, the mother cleans the room herself. Or instead of insisting that the child go to school, the father calls the principal's office and says, "Matthew isn't feeling well today." The truth, of course, is that Matthew is feeling lazy today, or Matthew didn't do his homework, or Matthew didn't study for his test.

All these things continue to insulate the youngster from responsibility. They corrupt the process of maturation, blocking the transfer of that parental-imposed control to self-imposed control.

Yes, the child is going to feel pain. Yes, riding a two-wheel bicycle for the first time entails a certain amount of risk.

But a healthy parent has to permit the child to fall. There is no other way to learn. Without risk, there is no meaningful success.

When a child is swallowed up in that overcoming or overprotective love, maturation grinds to a halt. Physiologically and chronologically, the child progresses normally, through adolescence and into early adulthood. But emotionally, that almost-grown-up person is still eight or nine or ten years old, completely unable to handle the stress of eighteen, nineteen, or twenty.

This breakdown of the family isn't limited to the United States. In fact, I have come across even more dramatic cases of it in some other parts of the developed world.

I remember back in the mid-1970s, in my travels as president of the World Federation of Therapeutic Communities, I visited our affiliate programs in Brazil. The condition of that country's young people struck me as truly alarming. The primary problem there wasn't drugs, although more recently that has become an increasing part of the equation. It was a breakdown of the family caused mainly by poverty and abandonment.

The very poor of Brazil are tucked off in the *favellas* of the great urban centers of Rio de Janeiro, São Paulo, and Recife. Back then, something like 10 percent of the nation's children under the age of fifteen were living on their own, having fallen completely out of the family—victims of this social disintegration, of this tragically pervasive abandonment.

That was more than fifteen years ago. Things have grown worse in Brazil in the intervening years. Currently, any visitor to the country—to Rio especially, but also the northern parts of Brazil—will see literally thousands of these young people on their own. They scrape by on the beaches and the back alleys, begging and hustling and robbing the tourists at noontime, almost under the eyes of the local police.

A statistic that is startling to me: In 1990, vigilantes killed 491 of these children because they represented a hazard to a healthy business climate and to public safety.

These castaway young people began living that way at ages as young as ten, eleven, or twelve. Now, they are emerging into their twenties and early thirties. And many of these former street kids have gotten into more serious crime, forming gangs of marauding thieves, wreaking havoc on the quality of life in some of South America's greatest cities, forcing society to pay the price of its long neglect.

That crisis in the Brazilian family was never addressed a decade or two ago. Now, it has turned into a major social emergency.

Around the world, the crisis of the family is wrapped in different packages. In some families, dire poverty is the primary cause. In others, abandonment is to blame—physical abandonment or emotional abandonment. This phenomenon of "throwaway children" has grown sadly common in the United States. Sometimes, the young people deal with their pain by literally running away. Other kids lash out, "getting back" at their perceived victimizers with violence, crime, or other hostile behavior.

Still others run away in their own minds, drowning their pain in alcohol or drugs. You see this not only in America but throughout the industrialized world—increasingly, even in the major cities of Third World countries. Malparenting and malnourishing are universal ills.

In Daytop, we confront this "baby problem." Our residents are young people who never grew up. They were constantly "running from," sometimes literally, more often chemically.

Our job is to teach them to mature, to catch up emotionally with their own chronological ages. We give them the tools to respond to stress. We run them through the family a second time. Whatever broke down the process the first time, we rebuild it and make it function again. Once that is accomplished, there is no more need for drugs.

That's why we always say that Daytop is not a drug-rehabilitation factory. We are a family. We're dealing with the young person in crisis. And while we are healing the young person, we are trying to heal the family as well.

This is what our Family Association is all about—and why it is so important to the success of Daytop.

We must never underestimate the potency of the family—both to heal and destroy itself. And let me tell you, the tragedies that have walked into Daytop over the years are enough to make you weep.

I remember one particular family, the O'Malleys. This goes back a few years, to when our Entry Unit was on Fortieth Street and Ninth Avenue, near the Port Authority Bus Terminal.

A young man showed up one day. His brother and sister brought him in. He was a barbiturate addict. A few days earlier, I had gotten a call from a priest friend who said he wanted to send the three of them down to see me. The younger brother, he said, was deeply into drugs. I said: "Sure, send them over."

It turned out that I had known the family back when I was a young priest. They used to come to church in the Bronx, where I was stationed at the time. The mother walked over and introduced herself one Sunday after Mass. Her husband was at Sloan Kettering, dying of cancer, she said. She wanted to know if I would pray for him.

I told her, "Sure, and I'll visit him, too, if you'd like me to." So I did, several times over the next week and a half. Each time I stopped by the hospital, she would be there. She was a remarkably stunning woman, beautiful inside and out, strong, gentle—the quintessence of a great lady.

I remember, a couple of times when I had stopped by the hospital, she excused herself halfway through the visit. She said she had to leave early. She had a baby in diapers at home.

Her name was Ilene O'Malley, and I'm sure I'll never forget her. The husband died quickly, and I remember visiting the house and seeing the three children, including the boy in diapers. They had to deal with great sadness, and the mother was a tower of faith and strength. She went out and got a job, and she did her best to press on.

And soon afterward, I was assigned to another parish, and I stopped seeing the O'Malleys. I knew the mother was working at a school somewhere, but we had completely lost touch.

And now this barbiturate addict sitting in front of me, Kevin O'Malley, had been that little kid in diapers. This was the older brother and sister, the family I had met all those years ago.

Barbiturates are one of the hardest drugs to shake. The drug gets an iron grip on the body. Barbiturate addicts get highly volatile when they're in need of a fix.

Kevin didn't remember our meeting, of course. But I told him my story about his mother and father and about meeting him as a young child. About halfway through he burst out crying. When he was thirteen or fourteen, he said, that beautiful mother of his had shriveled up and died of cancer, just as the father had.

As a matter of fact, Kevin told me, he took his first drugs the day after the funeral. He just couldn't cope with the loss of someone who was so central to his life, who was the focal point of all his love. He went downhill fast.

I got Kevin to call the Entry Unit. The person on telephone duty set up an appointment for Kevin at 8:30 the next morning.

The next day, I remember, was rainy. Kevin woke up surly, saying he wasn't sure he wanted to go. But the brother and the sister were insistent. They packed his clothes for him. And they told him to get in the car for the drive downtown.

But Kevin was growing increasingly agitated. He said he wasn't sure this was such a good idea. The whole notion of Daytop, he kept telling them, was a terrible, awful mistake. When they drove past Harlem, he tried to jump out of the car. He knew where he could score barbiturates there. But the brother kept talking to him, and by the time they got to Fortieth Street, Kevin had pretty much calmed down.

While the intake staff interviewed the brother and sister, a couple of the residents welcomed Kevin and brought him upstairs to see his room.

They were helping him unpack, and they were also going through his bags to make sure he hadn't brought any drugs with him.

When Kevin noticed this, he exploded in rage.

"Why are you doing that?" he demanded. "You have no right to do that. What's the matter? You don't trust me?"

"Of course not," one of the residents told him.

"Thank God no one trusted us when we came in," the other resident said. "We were dope fiends."

But Kevin persisted. "Don't look in my bag," he told them.

This went back and forth for another few seconds, when Kevin grabbed his bag and ran off toward the back stairway. He raced all the way down to the first floor and out onto Fortieth Street. He hailed a cab and directed the driver uptown.

The brother and sister were still upstairs being interviewed when the two residents came rushing in to tell what had just happened. They finished the interview, so we would have the information if Kevin decided to come back. Distraught, the brother and sister gathered up their things and headed back home to the Bronx.

By then, Kevin had already gotten back to the Bronx himself. He told the driver to pull over in front of a green two-story house, saying this is where he lived. He pretended to reach into his pocket for the cab fare. Instead, he snapped the door handle open. He grabbed his bag and leaped out the door. And he ran through one yard and into another. The driver tried running after him, but it was no use. This kid knew the neighborhood and was running awfully fast.

Kevin kept running until he got to the house of a boy named Peter. Kevin knew Peter would have pills to sell. He bought the downers and then walked to his girlfriend's house.

Elaine was her name. She was so happy to see him. She figured since he was going into Daytop, they wouldn't be together for months. Within an hour, they had picked up another couple and the four of them were driving through the side streets of the Bronx.

Elaine was sitting in the center of the front seat. Kevin was sitting to her right. The other girl was alone in the back. As they drove, Kevin was getting drowsy from the drugs. He leaned his head against Elaine's shoulder. This was nothing unusual. Kevin had always liked to do that, so she didn't pay this any particular mind.

They had been driving aimlessly around the northern Bronx for nearly an hour. After a while, Elaine noticed that Kevin's head was growing heavy. Her shoulder was beginning to ache. She nudged him with her shoulder and then poked him gently in the side. He didn't respond. When she lifted his head with her hand, it plopped right back down. It took her just another few seconds to realize that Kevin wasn't just sleeping. Something more was wrong.

She screamed at the driver: "Go to Jacobi Hospital."

When they pulled into the emergency entrance, Elaine opened the passenger door and climbed over Kevin. She didn't know he was already dead. She tried pulling him out of the seat, but he was too heavy. She pulled again, and she fell back onto the sidewalk. Kevin fell out on top of her.

True friends that drug addicts make, the driver flew into a panic. He threw the car back into gear, stepped on the gas and screeched out of the drive. He left Kevin and Elaine there on the sidewalk, she crying hysterically, he lying perfectly still.

Some nurse rushed over, but there was nothing they could do.

It was awful to preside at that funeral.

I couldn't help but remember Ilene O'Malley, that beautiful woman with those three promising kids.

I'd let one of them slip through my fingers. It took me weeks to get over that. I had let Kevin down. I had let his mother down.

Could we have helped Kevin at Daytop? The truth is I really don't know. Back at the seminary, they used to say that the Good Lord has plans. You can't play God. You don't win them all.

But even today, when I visit the Entry Center every Saturday and speak to the sixty-five young people who are there at any one time,

I start thinking again of Kevin. I thank God these other kids have a chance. They stand at the brink between life and self-destruction. I know they could fall either way. But if they have the strength—and if we have the strength—there is hope, I know. I thank the Lord at least these few have the opportunity to get their lives back together, to put their dreams back in place, to climb the hill together and see the sun rise.

PARENTING, THE HEART OF THE MATTER **14**

> *Even if time were not of the essence, the imperative would be much the same, for we cannot 'jump a generation' and* training for life as it is becoming *begins in, and reaches very far forward from the primary group of the home. The less of parents' work that has to be corrected, the quicker man moves ahead. The surer our aid to parents in preparing their young for life, the more geometrically expanding will be the resulting good to the greater number.*
>
> —Harry Stack Sullivan, M.D., *The Interpersonal Theory of Psychiatry*

One Wednesday night, I was working late in the office at Daytop headquarters. I always find it easier to get work done when the phones aren't ringing. It must have been almost nine o'clock by the time my desk was cleared and I was ready to head back up to the Bronx. I went down the back stairs onto the third floor and noticed that about a dozen of the parents were still there after meeting with their Daytop Family Association groups.

As I was walking past them, one couple got up and hurried over to introduce themselves. They said their names were Tony and Maria, and they had something they needed to tell me.

The man spoke uncomfortably, in a reserved sort of way. "Please excuse us," he said, "but we're a—we're people who feel a lot of emotion. And this is very emotional what happened to us."

They explained that their son, Frank, was in Daytop. The weekend before, he had just gotten his first permission for a family visit. He'd been with us for seven or eight months. That's about how long it usually takes before residents are permitted to begin seeing their families again.

Anyway, Tony and Maria had driven up on Sunday to see their

boy, who was at our house in Swan Lake in the Catskill Mountains. Then, they went on to describe what happened during that visit.

Their son, who had stolen from his father's wallet and sold his mother's jewelry to get money for drugs, who had told his parents he wanted to dance on their graves and said all the other hurtful things that addicts say to those who love them—that same son had run down the path and hugged his mother and said: "Mother, I love you. I'm sorry I broke your heart."

"That boy hasn't said anything like that in nine years," the father said. "And then he turned to me and said, 'Dad, I love you and I know you've been disappointed in me. I'm going to make it up to you.'"

The whole day up at Swan Lake had gone like that. Tony and Maria went through the long list of loving things their son had said and done. But toward the end of the day, Frank had turned to his mother and said, "Would you mind if Dad and I had a man-to-man talk for a minute?" Maria told them to go right ahead.

So father and son walked off down the path. After getting out of Maria's earshot, Frank said, "Dad, you are in Daytop family therapy. You understand what this means, right? When I graduate from Daytop, I can't work for you anymore."

"So I told him, 'Yes, son, I understand.'"

Now, hearing this story from Tony, I have to confess I didn't understand what he was getting at, especially by that last part. I asked him to explain.

"I have a butcher shop on Manhattan's Upper East Side, one of the richest residential neighborhoods in the world. I had the shop for a few years when a supermarket opened about a block north of me. About a year later, another supermarket opened up a block and a half to the south. I couldn't compete with the supermarkets in price—not with their volume. So I made a conscious decision. I had five children to support and a wife. So I've been putting my thumb on the scale and cheating my customers all these years.

Otherwise, I wouldn't survive. And I rationalized that this was all right. It was the best of a number of bad choices.

"Anyway, my son said to me, 'Dad, I hope you understand that I've learned in Daytop that honesty is the most important treasure that I have, and I can't let even a tiny speck of dishonesty into my life anymore. That's part of the reason that I ended up on drugs. I chose to be dishonest with myself and with the people who loved me and with everybody else. So I hope you understand, Dad. But I do love you.'

"I told the boy I understood, and tears filled my eyes. I knew the boy was right."

All this time Maria was nudging Tony to get on with the story. So I asked him: "I don't understand why you're telling me all this. Have you told your groups?"

Maria had one of those I-told-you-so looks on her face. I asked her whether she had told her group.

Both of them shook their heads no.

"We've told our groups everything about ourselves," Tony said. "They know everything. But we haven't been able to get up the courage to tell them about the butcher shop."

I was furious. I knew their groups would be furious, too. To hold back at Daytop is like keeping a little bit of poison inside yourself at a time you're supposed to be trying to get all the poison out. You can't be authentic and healthy until you get all the poison out. So I said to Tony and Maria, "Your groups are going to be very upset. But I want you to promise me that you're going to tell them next week. You'll feel better about it. Please tell the groups." They assured me they would.

Then, I headed down the stairs and out into the night. I didn't think about Tony and Maria again for another three months. They simply dropped from my memory. Then, one Wednesday, I found myself working late again. I headed down those same stairs on my way out of the building. I was walking across the foyer on the third floor when a couple came over to say hello.

I recognized them, but I wasn't sure from where. I asked them to refresh my memory. They reminded me of the conversation those many weeks before.

"Can we talk to you for a minute?" Maria asked.

"You are the couple that told me about your boy in Swan Lake. You had your visiting permission, and he told you he couldn't work for you anymore. So did you tell your groups?"

Tony said they had. "Let me tell you what happened, Father," he said. "I didn't sleep that whole week after we spoke. We have a close bond in our group. We really trust each other, and I had broken that bond. I hadn't been honest. So I couldn't sleep.

"Finally, Wednesday came around, and I went into my group. I was very nervous, and I literally got on my knees. It was very emotional because that's my nature. But I told them, and I pleaded with the group to please understand. I finally got that last rock out of my stomach, and it felt so good to get it out and be totally honest. The group was furious. They were yelling at me, and two of the men said they didn't buy that rationalization—that in order to support your family, you have to cheat.

"They shouted at me, 'Tony, you told us you and Maria had been fighting and you couldn't sleep over a number of years and you couldn't look your customers in the eye. That's no way to live. You have to be totally honest.' And two of the men mentioned that if the only way I am going to survive and be honest is to close the shop, that's what I am going to do and then come work for them."

Maria said just about the same thing happened in her group.

I didn't say anything, letting Tony and Maria know I was waiting to hear the rest of the story. You see, in Daytop, there is a commitment to change in all our groups. I wanted to know what Tony and Maria's commitment had been.

"Wait until you hear this," Tony said. "They told me that, when I opened the store the next morning, I had to tell all my customers the truth, the whole truth, every bit of it.

"I didn't sleep that night either. Maria and I went over to open the shop at seven thirty the next morning. We have a big glass door, and the lock is at the foot of the door. I was on my right knee unlocking the door when my first customer, Mrs. Mulhearn, arrived right behind us.

"I whispered 'good morning' to her and continued opening the door, thinking to myself: 'I don't know how I'm going to do this, but I have to do it.'

"So I stood up and opened the door, turned on the lights and held the door for Maria and Mrs. Mulhearn. When they got inside, I looked at Maria. She didn't say anything, but she nodded encouragingly. I took a deep swallow and told Mrs. Mulhearn the whole story. I told her I had rationalized that I had a license to cheat her. And I wasn't going to cheat anymore. I taught my boy to be a cheater and he went on drugs. Then, he taught me what honesty was. It's the greatest prize in life. It makes you free. I told all the rest of it too.

"You know I looked Mrs. Mulhearn in the eye for the very first time that morning. She had sweet green eyes, and they were filling up with tears. She reached over and hugged me. 'Tony and Maria,' she said, 'you are probably the most honest business people on all of Second Avenue.'

"That's what happened all day when I told my customers. Their eyes filled with tears and they hugged me and Maria. My customers went around and told other people the story, and those other people packed into the store just to hear it. We now have a real personal relationship with our customers, for the first time ever. We have a family on Second Avenue. We look out for each other. We visit each other in the hospital. We are sharing now. We never did that before. We were scared to. We never trusted each other. When I look at my customers now, I see beautiful people. I never saw that before.

"Maria and I have a new romance, too. It's built on honesty. When I go home at night now, for the first time, my head hits the pillow and I'm asleep in a flash. I have a sense of serenity in my life, brought about by my learning what the word *honesty* means. My boy did that for me, and I love him for it."

If you believe, as I do, that drug abuse is, in large part, a symptom of a deeper crisis in the family, then one conclusion follows logically from that belief: Part of the solution lies in healing the family itself.

That is why the Daytop Family Association exists.

When a young person comes to us, he or she is usually suffering the most obvious and most direct symptoms of that failed family. There are few options more self-destructive than drug addiction.

Elsewhere in that family, though, others are almost always suffering, as well.

If possible, those other family members must be brought into the process of recovery. For one thing, they can be a tremendous help in the addict's recovery. And at the same time, the family can almost always benefit from some parallel help of its own.

We do this by creating groups of family members—no more than ten to fifteen people. They meet once a week under the guidance of a trained group leader. In these groups, the family members are urged to speak openly and honestly about exactly what they are going through. This could involve feelings of shame or embarrassment or frustration about having a drug-addicted child. It could involve probing some of the deeper questions about how the various family members interact. It could involve coming to grips with the ways that family life contributed to the addict's addiction.

None of this is to absolve the addict of personal responsibility. At some point along the line, the addict had to push the needle into his own arm, or put the straw into her own nose, or suck the stem of a crack pipe with his or her own lips.

That said, however, families can help each other to construct a more healthy home life—if only they are given the tools.

Whatever the particular concerns of the family group, the usual Daytop rules about honesty and openness apply. And since everyone in the group has been through the problems of having a drug-addicted family member, the discussions can get extraordinarily intimate and deep.

The idea isn't to make judgments about one another. It's to benefit from the things that others have gone through—and, when possible, to extend a helping hand.

So when the conversation turns, for example, to the question of how a particular family contributed to a son's or a daughter's drug abuse, it isn't done for blaming. That accomplishes nothing. It is done for the purpose of understanding, so these unhealthy patterns can finally be left behind.

The Daytop Family Association, which had its first meeting back in 1966, has become well established over the years—an achievement due, in no small part, to the work of two towering individuals. Roxy and Berge Kalajian are Daytop parents and true visionaries. They came to us the way most parents do, because a drug-abusing child had left their family heartbroken.

They took their pain and despair, and they molded it into a new life as mentors in Daytop's family rescue mission. The Kalajians played a gigantic role in developing our philosophical system for teaching sound parenting. They remain mentors a quarter of a century later, traveling around the nation and the world, spreading our approach to model parenting.

At any one time, nearly sixteen hundred people participate actively. These aren't just silent names on a mailing list. They are people who attend weekly meetings at one of the ten Outreach Centers or our Midtown headquarters, people who recognize that they too have something to learn from Daytop and from each other. More than half of Daytop's residents have at least one relative attending meetings.

Most of the Family Association members have at least one relative in Daytop, although some have found that they continue to benefit from the association even after their relatives have finished with treatment. We welcome that.

Caring about a drug addict is not an easy thing. Addicts have a way of draining the people who care for them. After a while, the promises and the lies and the disappointments can take a terrible toll. What the Family Association tries to do is to take some of the techniques we have learned in the treatment of drug addicts and use them to help the addicts' families.

In the old days, we used to call this group the Daytop Parents Association. But it didn't take us long to figure out that the name was absurdly narrow. In today's world, the concept of family is much more complicated than that. Mom and dad aren't the only people who perform the traditional parenting role. And they aren't the only ones whose lives are thrown into turmoil by an addict's drug use.

Sometimes, it's a spouse or a grandparent or a brother or sister. It may be a gay lover or a live-in boyfriend or girlfriend.

Our job is not to decide whether each and every one of these relationships meets our notions of the traditional family. Traditionalists from the religious community might turn up their noses at some of the living arrangements that drug addicts end up in. But splitting these moral hairs is not Daytop's job. We are here for people as we find them. That is not an easy business, and we will take any help we can get.

And it turns out that the addict's family—however that word is defined—can be a tremendous help.

No one needs to be told that the family is under siege in America and other industrialized countries and that drug abuse is part of the fallout. There is also the destruction of the family by separation and divorce, the irresponsibility of parents creating throwaway children, and kids having kids of their own. Some of them, of course, are emotionally or physically abandoned. The whole secular culture places values on things rather than on right and wrong and on people and goals.

But provide families with the tools, and it is amazing the progress they can then achieve. The story of Tony and Maria is not an isolated one.

A big part of the process involves dealing with denial in the family. Just as we have to deal with denial on the community or the national level, the denial inside families is one of the major obstacles Daytop must face. When we are able to engage the family, we deal with people's natural unwillingness to look at the raw facts of drug abuse that are staring them in the face. This doesn't just involve the youngsters who are dying and their parents' inability to do anything about it. There are usually a whole host of other issues in the family life. When denial gives way, the release is marvelous. Positive things happen extraordinarily fast.

Before a child descends into the swamp of drug addiction, a whole array of signals has normally appeared, suggesting that the family is in trouble. Usually, those red lights have been signaling for a long period of time. But no one has recognized them.

Few people are equipped to notice these signs.

Those are the skills we teach in the Family Association. Perhaps Daytop is not ready to save the world. But we can save some families.

Save enough families—eventually you'll save the world.

Back in the early 1980s, an organization called the National Federation of Parents came onto the scene. In my view, the group had tremendous potential to improve the state of the American family. Uniting parents from across the country so they might trade useful information and advise each other in times of crisis: that was a terrific idea, long overdue. The federation sprang out of the experiences of a wonderful couple from Naples, Florida, Bill and Pat Barton, who found themselves facing the same challenges that millions of other parents have.

Their daughter was sinking deeper and deeper into marijuana use. Getting high had become the only thing in life she seemed to care about. Her friends, her family, her schoolwork—none of it seemed to hold the slightest interest anymore. When her parents tried to talk with her about the way she'd been acting, she lashed out, accusing them of secretly hating her guts.

Not surprisingly, the mother and father found this behavior alarming. They weren't quite sure what to do about it. But they knew they couldn't sit idly by.

So the Bartons began trying to motivate their community. They went to talk with the local police about this drug problem that had gotten a foothold among the city's young. They brought up the issue with the school authorities and with the people at city hall. Everyone seemed to listen with interest. And before long, these institutions were actually getting mobilized.

The school officials, for one, agreed that things had gotten a little out of hand. They arranged to have the school parking lots monitored in the morning and evening, and other gathering places as well. As an outgrowth of these discussions, the high school even adopted a dress code.

And all of this came from the efforts of one set of parents who had decided to get involved.

The Bartons figured they might as well set up a formal organization, and that's how the National Federation of Parents was born. The group really took off. Before long, they were expanding beyond Florida, setting up chapters in dozens of cities and towns. The effort generated some media interest, and the idea just seemed to hit a nerve. Nancy Reagan, who had only recently discovered the drug problem, got involved in a big and public way, talking up the organization and helping raise money to finance the group's expansion plans.

Then, just as quickly, the federation seemed to peter out. The chapters' leaders were unsure about what they should be doing. Mrs. Reagan lost interest. So did the other celebrity backers who had gathered around. Even the Bartons' vigor and enthusiasm wasn't enough. Despite the flash of interest, something about this admirable movement struck many people as a little off-key.

The basic problem, I think, was that nowhere in the programmatic goals was there anything about healing the family itself. All the attention was focused outside—on the community, the police, the schools, the media, and the big-name political patrons who were eager to bask in the federation's glow.

These social institutions could all stand improvement. But they are not the basic problem that the family faces today. Nor are they the front-line reason young people are turning to drugs.

The reason is the family's own failure to create a healthy environment of demanding love.

Drug addiction doesn't come from the school or from the police or from the public gathering places or even from the wrong crowd of friends, as so many parents want to believe. It comes from a breakdown in parenting, a failure in the family itself.

This is why at Daytop, our family-therapy groups look inward, as much as they look out—even more. The addict isn't the only one who needs healing. Almost inevitably, the family needs it, too.

In hindsight, the federation had some other limitations. The group's efforts were too narrowly focused on the concerns of the middle class. At the national conventions, for instance, minority faces were few and far between. And it is interesting that the group's main "problem drug," in the early years at least, was marijuana, which is primarily a middle-class phenomenon.

Still, the federation's inability to sustain itself is a great tragedy, I think. The idea of uniting parents in a nationwide movement is a genuinely sound one, with huge potential benefits for all of us. Unfortunately, this effort failed to have an adequate therapeutic base. They may have also gotten a little too captivated by the interest of all those celebrity-politicians.

In the end, I think, the federation never had time to learn a lesson that we at Daytop have come to know: the importance of clearly identifying your goals. You simply have to know what the targets are before you rush the troops into the field.

This is never quite as easy as it sounds. The problems of drug abuse are multifaceted, and each facet has to be confronted in a different way. The drug problem is really several problems in one—or more precisely, a continuum of problems, each blending into the next.

On the left of that continuum are the maximally disoriented drug users, many of whom have reached the point of no return. This is a terrible thing to say, but we cannot kid ourselves. Some people will never be saved. No family, no program will ever help them. They will probably never operate as productive members of society. They lack the very inclination to help themselves.

These are the calcified sociopaths. The sad reality is that for such people incarceration may be the only answer.

Moving across the continuum, the moderately disoriented drug users come next. They are like cliff-hangers, already in serious danger but with the possibility of rehabilitation and a return to family life. They may be heavy, heavy drug users, with hard addictions and repeated failures to break free. They may have already fallen away from their families and friends. They may have already tried to quit and failed. They may even be living in the gutter or in a jail cell. But somewhere deep inside them, a spark of hope still burns.

These are the people that residential drug treatment is best suited for. The road will not be easy. But if the will is buried somewhere deep inside them, we may well be able to help them dig it out and get on with their lives.

On the right side of the continuum is the third group, the minimally disoriented. They are the ones toying with mind-altering drugs in the locker rooms and video arcades and other places where young people congregate.

In a sense, they are the easiest of the three groups to reach. They are the most susceptible to the intelligent prevention campaigns (as distinct from the clumsy, overblown ones, which touch no one at all. Remember *Reefer Madness*?) These young people from the minimally disoriented group are the most open to antidrug role models and the entreaties of concerned relatives and friends. On the treatment side, they can be motivated with the less-dire outpatient approaches, the programs like Daytop Outreach.

Unfortunately, groups like the National Federation of Parents—and Mrs. Reagan, their patron—targeted only the continuum's far right side. Their campaigns could not possibly have had an impact on anyone but the least disoriented young. This was easy, and it hit close to home. Many of these young people, after all, were children of the middle class. It's lovely to be able to see rosy-cheeked young people who still could smile in front of a flapping American flag.

But by and large, they aren't the drug users who cause the problems that society worries about.

The real trouble comes from the ones in the middle and on the left side of that continuum—the moderately and severely disoriented addicts. They are the ones who have fallen out of the family, who have sought to self-medicate their pain with drugs. They are trying to make their way through life crises that are unbearable, and they lash out in socially destructive ways.

They are the ones, in other words, who will mug you on your way home at night, or hold up the corner liquor store.

What thirty years at Daytop have taught us is no one answer is right for all three groups. That is why we have residential and outpatient treatment, and that is why we never promise to succeed with everyone.

That would be as silly as telling a hard-core drug addict to "Just say no."

I remember one mother who was doing her best to raise a teenage boy in a changing neighborhood in the Bronx. Drugs were everywhere in that community, sold in the open on street corners, even dealt over the counter of the local bodega.

Sheila Nolan was her name. Her husband, Neil, was a hard-working proprietor of a corner grocery. She had watched drugs take over the area and destroy the children of so many neighbors she could not possibly keep count.

But Sheila was not one to think of herself as a victim. She just vowed she would do whatever she could—*whatever,* she told herself—to make sure young Patrick had every chance.

So she tried to keep him busy. And she worked with her husband at the grocery to help provide some of the little extras for her family. The long hours often left her tired at night. But she always made a special effort to keep the lines of family communication open, and she figured things were going pretty well.

One morning, though, while cleaning Patrick's room, she came across something that made her heart almost stop: two small glassine envelopes with white powder inside.

"Drugs," she thought immediately. But she wasn't really sure.

In a panic, she ran out of the apartment with the envelopes and right over to the Fifty-second Precinct.

But she didn't even get inside. She saw a squad car parked out front, with two officers just sitting there, and she walked up to the passenger window.

"I'm sorry to disturb you," she said, "but can I ask you a question?"

Both cops had bored looks on their faces, but simultaneously they nodded yes.

She thrust her right arm into the squad car, holding the envelopes about halfway between the two cops. "I found these in my son's drawer," she said. "Can you tell me what they are?"

The officer in the driver's seat took the bags. He pulled one of them open and wet the index finger on his left hand. He dipped his finger into the powder and then touched the finger to his tongue.

"How old is your son?" he asked her.

"He's seventeen."

"Where do you live?" the cop asked.

"On the Concourse."

"An apartment building?" She nodded. "How high is it?"

This struck her as an odd question. But she answered anyway. "It's six stories. What do you mean?"

"Listen to me a second," the officer said. "If I were you, I'd go home and I'd take that boy up to the roof of your building. I'd walk him right up near the edge, and then I'd push him off."

The mother didn't say a word. A terrible look just flashed across her face. She snatched back the envelopes from the officer and, crying, she ran all the way home.

She never did take her son up to the roof. Instead, when she got back to the apartment, she started dialing the telephone. She called a priest she knew, Father Ned Murphy, who ran a program for homeless men, and told him about what she had found. He put her in touch with Daytop.

It took a while to get Patrick to agree to treatment. When she confronted him, he admitted he'd been using heroin for more than a year. He insisted, though, he wasn't addicted. Slowly though, he acknowledged that the habit was getting expensive and his life was slipping out of control.

After several weeks of back and forth, Patrick agreed to give Daytop a try.

He blossomed in treatment. And Sheila came regularly to Family Association meetings, bringing Neil with her. She found them tremendously valuable to her. She learned things about her family—and ways of dealing more effectively with her son.

She had never realized, she told her group one night, how in her desire to protect her child she had really helped prevent him from growing up.

Patrick has been clean now for more than five years. He graduated from Daytop and is now running the grocery store on his own.

Recently, I got a letter from Sheila. She said she could hardly believe how the time had flown.

"That Saturday when I found the drugs in Patrick's room," she wrote, "I was devastated. I was even more devastated when I went up to the precinct to find out what was in those bags. 'Your son is better off dead.' Could a mother be told anything more terrible than that?

"That all seems so long ago. It is only five years, I know. But we've all come so far.

"Patrick is doing wonderfully. I just wish I had the words to express how much I learned from the other parents who were in my group.

"I'll never forget my first Family Association meeting and how scared I was. I was so filled with denial. But the love and support I got there and the strength to carry forward—how blessed I was! I learned to give healthy love to my son. I discovered how to say no. I came to understand that no matter how alone I felt, I was really never alone. Whatever my problems, other people had dealt with them before—even more severe ones. For me, that is where the strength came from."

SHADOWBOXING WITH ADDICTION 15

> *The most rapid possible liquidation of adolescent delin-*
> *quency and institution of a program to prevent its recur-*
> *rence is thus becoming a matter of national security. If we*
> *have not been interested in doing this job for moral reasons,*
> *we are going to be compelled to do it for the sheer sake of*
> *survival. So the sooner we get going the better. We are coming*
> *up to the time when juvenile delinquency will be a luxury*
> *which we no longer can afford. There is no question but*
> *that we can end it. But the rehabilitation of the shook-up*
> *generation is going to require some changes in us as well*
> *as in the adolescents.*
>
> —Harrison E. Salisbury, *The Shook-up Generation*

Denial.

When someone uses that word in connection with drugs, a single image often springs to mind: that of a young addict, trying to talk his way out of trouble.

"Me? No way, Mom. I would never use that stuff."

"Those aren't my drugs. Honest, Officer. I was just holding the bag for my friend."

"A problem? Not me. I can stop anytime I want to."

Anyone who spends time around drug addicts is well acquainted with that kind of denial. We hear it at Daytop every time new residents arrive, before they've had a chance to learn our code of utter honesty.

But there is another kind of denial out there. In many respects it is far more pernicious than the junkie's predictable lies—and a bigger obstacle to the mission of Daytop. This is denial by society, the amazing ability of otherwise savvy people to hide their eyes from the reality of drugs. It is a phenomenally powerful force in our world today.

Societal denial comes in many varieties: The parents who want to believe that drugs exist only in some other neighborhood. The school authorities who are absolutely convinced that none of their students could be involved. The clergymen who say, "This is not a matter for the pulpit. It's a matter for the police." And the politicians, at all levels of government, who see the drug issue not as an opportunity to rescue human beings but as an easy stage to pander on.

This kind of denial has a long and ignoble history. Its reach extends from the bottom of society to the top. It is the biggest threat that our movement faces. This has been true from the beginning. It remains true today.

Just about every single time that Daytop has sought to open a new facility, we have come face to face with this denial.

It barely seems to matter where we go. Rich neighborhood, poor neighborhood, big city, small town. It's the same story everywhere. The local residents find out that a drug-treatment program is moving into the community. They respond with angry cries of "Go away!" And we find ourselves fighting with the very people we have come to serve.

They deny their community has a drug problem.

They say the problem's not nearly as bad as it obviously is.

They say Daytop will only make things worse.

They say our residents will pose a horrible threat to their neighborhood.

Or they say we will send their property values through the floor.

The truth is that all this fear and anger is really just a symptom of the denial. Its grip is so strong, though, that some people will say anything they can think of to try to keep us out.

They rarely succeed. But the hurdles they place in our way—the hostile meetings, the high-priced court battles, the hardball poli-

ticking—have become a predictable hindrance to the t
drug addicts everywhere.

At Daytop, we got a rude and early introduction to tl
denial, as we were opening our first house on Staten Is
years ago. We didn't make any official announcements.
spread briskly about our plans—or, as the local versio
about the "dangerous drug addicts" who would soon be
in. Our neighbors erupted in outrage. Their supercharged r
went on into the evening. They threw rocks and bottles
residents and staff. They demanded that the local politica
sentatives find a way to run us off the island.

They wanted to believe that drugs were somebody else's
lem. They were deeply embedded in denial. So they saw [
as a threatening intruder, ready to wreck the island's tranqu
of life. The neighbors were worried about the safety of their
dren. They were anxious about the value of their homes. They
sure that we were about to corrupt the things they held most (

The hidden truth, of course, was that Staten Island in the e
1960s, like a lot of places, had its problems with drugs. Local l
were shooting dope out on the beach at night. Junkies were bri
ing in heroin from Brooklyn and selling it at jacked-up prices ri
outside the St. George Ferry Terminal.

In fact, Daytop was not the thing that threatened Staten Islande
Daytop was the beginning of an answer to a threat that was alread
in their midst. But none of this jibed with the image of middle
class Staten Island. It didn't matter that some of Daytop's earl
residents had actually grown up in the neighborhood. Nor did i
matter that Daytop offered a much needed glimmer of hope. Far
better to attack the bearer of the unwelcome news.

To be fair to our early opponents, Daytop had absolutely no track
record at that point. We talked a pretty good game, I think. We told
our neighbors not to worry. We told them our intentions were
pure. But what reason did they have to believe anything we said?

In the years since then, we have built up a glowing track record

of smooth operation and accomplishment. We've helped more than seventy thousand addicts overcome the ravages of drugs, and we've done it without a single incident around our centers to justify the neighbors' fears.

We have eight big Daytop houses in Upstate New York now, and ten drop-in centers in the metropolitan area. And that doesn't even include our headquarters building in midtown Manhattan, our Entry Unit in Queens, our training center in Milford, Pennsylvania, and the new Daytop Villages that have opened in Texas and California and Florida and overseas.

At each location, we take great pains to be a good neighbor. All our properties are immaculately kept—by the residents, of course. In several of the low-income neighborhoods where we have facilities, our buildings have helped to stabilize deteriorating blocks. In the middle-class areas, we have proven ourselves time and again.

Especially during Re-entry, Daytop residents are expected to become involved in the community in a productive, positive manner. This means patronizing local merchants, participating in community projects, contributing in various other socially useful ways.

Even on the financial balance sheet the results have been positive at every step. Despite the fears that we would wreck local property values, this has never turned out to be the case. If anything, we have enhanced the neighborhoods we have moved into, after the initial furor died down.

But you know what?

None of this seems to have mellowed our opponents or loosened the powerful grip of denial.

Still, almost every time we seek to open a new Daytop facility, it's Staten Island all over again. Almost without exception, our plans generate tremendous opposition. What a sad commentary on the state of our world!

In the end, thankfully, we have almost always been able to convert the neighbors. Time after time, our staunchest opponents have become our staunchest friends. They're not bad people, really.

They're just caught up in that cycle of denial. I only wish we could figure out some way to carry the lessons of one community into the next place Daytop goes. It would make things so much easier for us and for them.

Every time I think about this subject, my mind wanders back to two evenings on Staten Island, ten years apart.

The first was that memorable evening at our inaugural Staten Island Center when a few hundred enraged neighbors marched on the new Daytop House. The anger in their eyes wasn't so different from what you might expect at a Ku Klux Klan rally in the Old South. If things had turned out just a little differently, I firmly believe our neighbors could have burned us down.

The protest that night was led by an off-duty New York City policeman, who outscreamed everyone else who was there. He had his nine-year-old with him, and the boy clenched his Dad's hand. Two things were obvious about this duo. The little guy was frightened out of his skin. And Dad was very, very drunk. We invited the howling mob to come inside and meet the frightened Daytop residents. Almost half took us up on the offer and stayed with us for hours, visibly touched by the Daytop residents. The rest of the mob resorted to violence, smashing windows and attacking automobiles. It was a horrible evening all around—one, by the way, that won for Daytop new friends all over New York, in the media and across the community.

But the importance of that night pales in comparison to what happened a decade later, when we tried to open an Outreach Center in Staten Island's West Brighton neighborhood. All the usual canards about outsiders in the community no longer held true: This was a daycare center just for young Staten Islanders, every one of whom would go home to their families at night. Still, the public meeting was filled with rage and rancor. Very few of the opponents cared to hear our words. We were near churches, schools, centers for the aged, they complained. We were a menace, they said. When we countered that their own active street addicts were the real threat, they shouted us down.

Then, suddenly a man stood up in the center of the room. He seemed gripped with a moving story to tell. He pleaded to be heard. "Please, listen," he said. "Please hear me."

And he began. "I am a New York City police officer," he said. "Ten years ago, I led a march to destroy the first Daytop in Tottenville. I was drunk that night. I was always drunk. I refused to face that problem. My marriage was breaking up. My kids were terrified of me. My life was a mess. That night at Daytop, I had my nine-year-old son with me. I am ashamed to tell you that my alcoholism and family abuse drove him to drugs. He entered Daytop and got his life back together. In Daytop's wonderful family-therapy group, I came to grips with my alcoholism. Haven't had a drink in two years. My son is doing very well—no drugs in two years also. My family is back together. All this is made possible by Daytop. Thank God for Daytop. How stupid I was that terrible night! How ashamed I am to talk about this now! But please, please, don't repeat my mistake. Don't fight Daytop. Welcome Daytop. It can save your child and family, too."

His dramatic words hung over the room. No one dared to speak. That particular fight was over.

What makes this denial even sadder is the role played by the people who pretend to be our leaders.

The minute the subject of drug treatment arises, the self-promoting politicians begin hovering, sniffing around for an easy place to grandstand, ready to trade the future of their young constituents for a few points in the polls.

This is probably the most revolting aspect of all my work—watching these grown men and women who are elected to seek out the well-being of their communities, playing to the bleachers instead.

Twist the truth?

You bet.

Play to the base emotions?

If it works, why not?

Scapegoat the weakest among us?

Sure, whatever it takes. The young people of their districts may be in great travail. But why worry? Most of them don't even vote.

I remember one particular member of the New York State Assembly, who came from Staten Island and headed the important committee on mental health. For many years, that panel handled funding for drug programs across New York State, until a separate drug-abuse committee was set up.

This woman traveled all over the state, championing the cause of drug treatment. Then, we decided to open a new center in Staten Island, and she fought us every inch of the way. She claimed we had tried to sneak into her neighborhood. She wasn't against Daytop, she insisted, nor was she against the idea of drug treatment. She was just upset that we had not made a public announcement in advance about our plans.

We explained to her that we were not trying to hide anything from anyone. We wanted to let our immediate neighbors know first about what we had planned. That's why we sent out small teams of Daytop staff and residents, door to door, to visit with the local merchants and clergymen and school officials. Daytop, after all, was still an unknown quantity to many of them. This was all leading up to the public announcement, which we made exactly as planned.

The legislator brushed aside our explanations and continued her bitter (though ultimately unsuccessful) fight to keep us out.

Ten years later, when we needed more room and moved that center to a different neighborhood on Staten Island, we hoped to learn from our unpleasant experience the first time out. So we reversed the process. We made the public announcement first, and then we sent the teams around to visit with the people in the neighborhood.

But the same legislator led the charge against us again, and just as bitterly as before.

She was outraged, she said, that we had the nerve to make a public announcement without discussing our plans first with her and other members of the community. This was the height of arrogance, she told me on the phone.

So I paid a call on her to ask what exactly we should have done.

I minced no words when she showed me into her office and invited me to sit down.

"You're an eloquent defender of our cause, and we appreciate that," I told her. "Except on Staten Island. Here, you are a demagogue. You are our most strident foe. We've tried it both ways. You didn't like either one of them. Can you suggest another way we should go about dealing with the political leaders on Staten Island?"

She said something about special conditions and something else about different communities having different needs. But she didn't really have an answer to my questions—except to say how busy she was and to suggest firmly that I should be on my way.

There is no reason to pretend. Reactions such as these are terribly frustrating. Political survival often takes priority over kids. Thankfully, this attitude hasn't stopped us from doing our work. In spite of this leadership vacuum and the consistently grotesque performance of the local politicians, we have eased the anguish of more than nine thousand families on Staten Island and the lives of a like number of kids. These are children, I firmly believe, who would be in jail cells or on slabs in a morgue somewhere if it weren't for our determination to open against all odds. We've had to confront all types of opposition, running the gamut from genuine fear about safety and property values to the pure skullduggery of cynical politicians.

We believe we owe that first group a careful response. The second group, unfortunately, is beyond our reach. I'm sure that as long as the flags of democracy prevail—and I hope they do, with some improvement—we will have to put up with sickening manipulation like that.

Thankfully, Daytop has grown strong enough to win many—though not all—of these fights. Some of the newer treatment programs, unfortunately, even those we helped to build, are not yet this far along.

It is just maddening they get so little help from the politicians. City councilmen and state legislators all across America are scandalously unwilling to put their own prestige behind treatment, even those politicians who understand personally how important treatment is.

The simple truth is that every program has to be located somewhere. And everywhere is someone's backyard.

They're just politicians, people have tried to tell me over the years. What can you expect? Everybody knows what it takes to get elected to public office today—the big campaign contributions, the backroom deals, the daily compromises, the bowing to pressure from this or that interest group. No wonder the leaders we elect so seldom live up to the decency we have every right to expect.

Well, I'm still hoping. And in fact, a few high-minded political leaders do appear on the public stage from time to time. But how do we explain our weak-kneed educators and clergymen, the people at the top of our great moral institutions? They are the ones who are expected to rise above selfish concerns and promote higher values, the ones who are supposed to help us tell the difference between right and wrong. Where are they on the drug question? Why are they so paralyzed by denial?

I'll never forget a telephone call I got one afternoon from the principal of a prestigious Catholic girls high school in the heart of Manhattan. When I picked up the phone, the principal, a woman I knew reasonably well, had panic in her voice.

"It's terrible," she said, her voice quaking as she spoke. "Two girls in our senior class are going to be arrested this afternoon for distributing drugs. The sergeant just called to warn me. He said they sold drugs to an undercover police officer."

She was right. This was not good news. But she said she was trying to manage the situation as well as she could. "I think I've taken all the correct steps so far," she told me.

"Like what?" I asked her.

"Well," she said, "I asked the sergeant if the girls could go home first and change out of their school uniforms. He said that would be okay. And I asked him if the officers would, please, let the girls be arrested across the street and not on the school grounds. He said that would be all right, too. That's the way it's supposed to happen. We'll try to spare the school's image as much as we can."

An understandable reaction, I suppose. But just about as wrong as can be.

The principal was wrapped up in denial. Her answer to drugs was to hide. Image was paramount. You could hear the unstated fear in her voice: "Would parents stop sending their daughters to that school with the drugs?" She was more worried about the school's reputation than about what was happening to two of her students and what might happen in the future to the other girls.

She had no idea about how counterproductive her approach to the problem was.

"Tell you what," I said to her. "Leave the girls in their school uniforms. Let the narcotics cops take them right out of class. Then, call a general assembly and admit the school has a problem. Concede that your school is part of the prevailing anguish of the young. Mobilize yourselves to deal with it. Get the teachers and the students involved in confronting the problem. We'll be there to help you every step of the way."

That is what they did. Although I wouldn't say it eliminated the school's drug problem, it did bring the situation out in the open and permit the people most affected to get involved in finding solutions—instead of hiding from the challenge of being a caring school.

This was a few years ago, and I'm happy to say, marked improvements have been made since then—not just at this school but at schools across the country. Some have set up awareness groups. Others invite people from Daytop and our sister treatment programs to speak with their students. These in-school prevention programs are nowhere near enough to solve the drug problem in America. But at least they are a positive force, pushing our young people in the right direction. Some schools have begun responding to the life crises that propel kids toward drugs and have stopped minimizing the problems that this creates. Thankfully, schools are not so quick today simply to expel a student who is involved with drugs, relieved that they have avoided an embarrassment and confident that the problem has, therefore, been eliminated.

Many of our churches and temples haven't moved even that far.

I remember when we first opened on Staten Island, some of the most virulent opposition to our plans came from the local Catholic parish. At the time, the church had some valiant young priests, voices crying in the wilderness, who were touching the daily pain of families anguished by drugs. But their number was far too small.

As a matter of fact, the most threatening mob that ever marched on a Daytop house came from the community center of that particular parish. And three decades later not so much has changed. When we opened the day-care center just for Staten Island kids and I asked the local vicar whether he would come out foursquare for the kids of Staten Island who had a need for treatment, he said he couldn't. The local parish opposed us, he explained. If the people were against it, he said, there was no way the vicar could be a public friend of ours.

Imagine that: questions of right and wrong being put to a public plebiscite—by a Catholic parish that desperately needed to be educated about concern for its young! Thirty-seven percent of area families were headed by just one parent, and drugs were running through the community like a rip tide! And the church leaders stand aside and let it all happen! Not a very encouraging sight.

In no other area that I know of does the church teach by plebiscite. Divorce? Birth control? Abortion? I don't remember the church waiting for poll results before articulating the teachings on those subjects. Why drugs?

We teach moral values. We teach concern. We teach charity and love for one another and the sanctity of human life. Yet when it comes to the embarrassing problems associated with drug use, what we get from the pulpit—and Catholics are not alone here—is mass abdication of responsibility. We see a total lack of leadership. Instead, we get concern for property values in a particular neighborhood instead of the human values of its kids.

Today at least we have a vanguard of young and dedicated clergy and lay people of all faiths who have banded together to remove the blinders from their eyes and to devote their energies to doing something about this terrible crisis.

What is frustrating is how much work they have ahead of them.

Denial by our leaders, denial by our neighbors—these are awesome forces to fight against. Add in the denial so many of us practice ourselves. You can see why the progress against drugs is made one painful inch at a time.

There's a cardinal rule in journalism: If you want to understand what's going on, follow the money. It will tell you what your society really cares about.

When it comes to drugs, "getting tough" is what Washington and the local governments are interested in. That's where the overwhelming majority of the money goes.

Being tough on drugs is a good thing, of course. No one is tougher on drugs than Daytop. One day at one of our houses is ample proof of that. Far too often, though, it's exactly the wrong kind of toughness that our governments are eager to support.

Building prisons, for one thing. And creating new paramilitary police units. There's a deluge of government funding for those initiatives, while treatment programs like Daytop must eke by on crumbs.

Today, America has twice as many prosecutors as in 1980. We also have twice as many people serving time in prison. In fact, the United States keeps more people behind bars—per capita and in absolute numbers—than any other country in the world. More than China. More than the Soviet Union. More than South Africa.

And what has this done to eradicate drug abuse? Not an awful lot. If anything, the drug culture inside prison is more pervasive than on the street. At the same time, all these prosecutors and prison beds have been just as ineffective at getting crime off the streets. The crime rate remains frighteningly high—especially the rate of violent crimes like rape, robbery, murder, and assault. These numbers rise and fall a little from time to time. But plainly, all the law enforcement in the world isn't making the crime go away.

John Chancellor, the veteran NBC newsman, pointed out these facts recently at the inauguration of the new Daytop center outside Dallas. Chancellor knows a thing or two about drugs—and not just from his television work. He had a son who graduated from Daytop.

"We live in this country in what I call a culture of false toughness," Chancellor said. "We see it in the big money-making movies and in the prime-time TV shows about cops or vigilantes who take the law into their own hands. We see the culture of false toughness in some of our politicians, who act as though the only answer to society's problems is to lock up as many miscreants as possible. Tough talk is cheap in every country, and it is also politically popular."

The problem, in Chancellor's view, is that America has chosen the simpleminded toughness of police and prosecutors over a kind of toughness that is harder to explain but really works: the toughness of treatment. "What we have too often done, in plain language,"

Chancellor said, "is to ask the cops to solve societal problems that are beyond the capacity of the cops to solve.

"Toughness doesn't come out of the barrel of a gun, and you don't find it in a prison cell. Toughness means sticking with the program, staying the course, doing the job. It doesn't mean showing off, and it doesn't mean living in a culture of false toughness."

People who watch television will know this concept as the gospel of Frank Perdue: "It takes a tough man to make a tender chicken." It applies to people just as well.

Funding decisions are not the only way that Washington's denial asserts itself. It starts even before the money is doled out, even before the first shot is fired in the various permutations of our so-called national War on Drugs.

It starts with the gathering of statistics, a science that is practiced in this area with considerable sleight of hand.

Thirty years ago, the U.S. government, in an official study, declared the number of heroin addicts in the country to be half a million. No one knew the actual number. The estimate was arrived at by counting the number of treatment slots, interviewing social workers, and taking some wild guesses. But 500,000 was a nice round number. It was widely accepted, and it stuck.

For more than a quarter century, it has not been adjusted again.

We went through the 1960s, the 1970s, the 1980s. The drug culture ebbed and flowed. New drugs grew in popularity. Later, other drugs took their places. But as far as the federal government was concerned, heroin use was as constant as the North Star—500,000, still.

And vital policy decisions were actually made on the basis of this.

Even now, similarly contrived surveys appear all the time—usually promoting a particular political agenda. They will "prove" a downward trend, or a corner turned, or light at the end of some tunnel. These clichéd images are then bandied about in the game of politics for the sake of partisan edge.

That's what the Bush administration drug czar, William Bennett, did just before he resigned. He trotted out a set of putative statistics, announced a corner had been turned, and declared that his job at last was done.

Meanwhile, just as many addicts were dying from overdoses. Just as many crack babies were being born. Just as much heroin and cocaine was on American streets. And sadly, just as little attention was being shown to the few promising answers to drug abuse.

This is nothing new. I remember some years ago, when the national government put out a survey that indicated that the sale of records of drug-oriented rock groups had dropped markedly. Therefore, the government-paid researchers concluded, young people were showing less and less interest in drugs.

At this particular time, we had that whole wave of kids on roller skates with Sony Walkmans strapped to their belts and headphones pressed against their ears.

They were listening to the same, drug-oriented rock music they always had. Only now, they were buying it on cassette. Watch out for the next chapter in this survey. Compact disks have all but taken over the recorded-music business. How long can it be until someone notices a decline in cassette sales and attributes it to some new corner that has been turned against drugs?

Here's another example: Every year, the federal government conducts an extensive poll of high school seniors, questioning them about drugs and other topics. Periodically, the survey will reveal a drop in drug use.

But what exactly does this mean? The whole survey flies in the face of a sad reality: the largest percentage of young drug addicts drop out of school well before senior year.

That's why Daytop has opened high schools in its treatment centers. Most serious young drug addicts don't hang around school long enough to graduate. So when the government goes into the high schools and polls seniors about their drug use, they are the ones who are left, the ones who aren't usually as deeply into drugs.

What kind of barometer is that? What does it tell us about our national problem? The government knows about these flaws in its numbers. I am certain of that. I have discussed the matter with officials in Washington at the highest levels. But it's a useful manipulation, a means of showing progress where progress is notoriously difficult to find. So it continues, year after year.

This manipulation of the reality of drug abuse is a constantly recurring theme. What is so saddening is that the government, which should be interested in the facts and the future of our young people, is so quick to wink. Political hide is considered a more valuable commodity than the truth about the lives of our young. As long as those are our priorities, the manipulation will continue, and the national picture of drug abuse will remain an unbelievable caricature.

All this denial—by our local political leaders, by our most trusted institutions, by our national government—does terrible damage to the cause of healing America. Those of us who have dedicated our lives to this struggle, fight against it every day.

But there is one other variety of denial that, at times, can be even more potent than the other three combined. It is also the one kind of denial that most of us could wake up one morning and actually do something about.

That is the denial in our own families.

Most parents are extremely slow to recognize when the problem of drugs has arrived on their own doorstep.

Everyone wants to think it's the neighbor's boy or the neighbor's girl down the street—or better yet, those anonymous kids in the projects or the young hoodlums from the other side of the tracks.

Some parents go to extraordinary lengths to keep up the facade of denial.

The daughter gets arrested? Well, she was just holding someone else's bag.

Drugs turn up in the son's bedroom? Well, one of his friends must have left them there.

This well-orchestrated denial, which can sometimes go on for years, usually adds up to one basic reflex: "I can't stand to admit I have failed as a parent. I don't want to damage the public image of my family while my child is dying in front of my eyes. So I refuse to see the problem myself."

I remember back when I was first getting into this business, a television anchorman came to see me one day. He had a son who was a drug addict, and as it happens the boy had been arrested for a string of burglaries and had recently gone to jail.

Well, the father was so swept up with his own public image that he couldn't stand to face the obvious facts. He told me the police had misunderstood the boy. His son wasn't a bad kid, the father assured me. He had just gotten in with the wrong crowd of friends.

I smiled as he finished the story. This was obviously not the reaction he was looking for, and his face grew quickly flushed with anger.

"What are you smiling about?" he asked tersely.

I didn't answer the question directly. "Did you come here for advice?" I asked him.

"Yes," he said tentatively.

"Here's what I would do," I told him. "Do not visit him in jail."

He interrupted me right there. "I was going up there today."

"Don't visit him at all," I repeated myself. "Leave him in jail. Don't bring him anything. Don't call. Don't write. Don't send him any packages. Don't pay any visits at all."

He was looking at me blankly.

"Then, after he's been in for a couple of weeks and he's had a good long time to stare through the bars and think about where his life is heading, we'll send a Daytop team up to interview him. I predict that he'll be like a ripe apple for treatment. But if you go up there and visit him now, he'll find a way to con you and get your support for the things he's doing, and no one—not you, not us, or anyone else—will make any progress with that son of yours."

The anchorman, of course, disregarded everything I said. He went to see his son that afternoon. The child turned on his woe-is-me charm. The father gave him the approval and support that all but guaranteed the boy would learn nothing from his brief time in jail. As soon as the judge set bail, the father put up the money and got the boy out.

The only bright spot was the boy's mother. She couldn't prevail upon the father. But she recognized the signs of trouble and began attending the meetings of one of our family groups. She learned a little about what the problem was. Unfortunately, it took another crisis to open her husband's mind.

It was about three months later that her husband called on me again.

He appeared more desperate this time. He said he had gotten a call from his son, whom he hadn't seen in weeks. The boy was coming to the house in a couple of hours, he said. He had met a girl and he was moving into her apartment. The boy sounded drugged up when he called. He put the girl on the phone to say hello. She sounded as stoned as he did.

They were coming to the house in her car to move his things out.

"What do you think I should do?" the man asked me.

"Are you gonna follow my advice this time?"

He nodded. "What is it?"

"When the boy comes, remind him that he has stolen from your house, forged checks on your account, and lied to you a hundred times to get money. Tell him that you want him to leave. Chances are, he'll ignore you. He'll march right upstairs to his bedroom and begin moving out his old things. You call the police. Have him arrested. It's the most loving thing you can do."

The anchorman looked as though he had just been kicked in the teeth. "Really?" he said.

"Yes," I told him. "And leave him in jail this time. In a couple of weeks, we'll send someone over to interview him. Don't you go over there at all. Have your wife go. She understands the difference between love and blanket approval. You aren't at that point yet."

This time, the father was ready. The cops came to the house. They arrested the boy. The judge set bail again. It was a little higher this time, though the anchorman could easily have afforded it. But he didn't put up the cash. The boy sat in the Westchester County Jail for about three weeks, and then we sent someone over to interview him.

By then, he was ready for treatment. He came into Daytop, and he did very well.

I wouldn't say we ever entirely won over the father. He could never get out from under the sway his own image had over him. He never came to the Daytop family meetings, although the mother came every week. And most important of all, their son today lives a drug-free life.

THE MANDATE TO RECONCILE 16

> *Man has a great need to know whether it is worthwhile
> to be born, to live, to struggle, to suffer and to die—and
> whether it is worthwhile to commit oneself to some ideal
> superior to material and contingent interests—whether, in
> a word, there is a WHY that justifies his earthly existence....*
>
> *Unfortunately, in our age scientific rationalism and the
> structure of industrial society, which is characterized by the
> iron law of production and consumption, have created a
> state of mind that is fixed on a plan of temporal and earthly
> values, which deprive human life of all transcendental sig-
> nificance....*
>
> *This, then, is the essential problem: giving a* meaning *to
> the human being, to his choices, to his life and to his journey.*
>
> —Pope John Paul II, Castel Gandolfo, Italy, August 5, 1979

I was just a boy of eight when my parents decided to take me on a long automobile trip. This was the summer of 1932, and I can still remember it vividly: the three of us piling into our trusty old Buick, heading off into a part of the country that I had never seen and that my parents didn't know well. We were going south, as far as New Orleans. To a child who had spent his entire life in the suburbs of New York City, we might as well have been going to the other side of the Earth.

We had a brief stop for food in Tuscaloosa, Alabama, a quiet town with immaculate streets and fastidious white-porch houses. I couldn't believe how neat and well tended everything was. But I was far more taken aback by an incident that unfolded right before my eight-year-old eyes, just after we had finished lunch. Apparently, the sidewalks of Tuscaloosa back then were reserved for the town's white citizens. Blacks were expected to walk in the gutter. Racial prejudice was a fact of life all over the United States in the 1930s.

But the openness of this southern variety came as quite a shock to this northern boy.

Suddenly, a red-and-white sheriff's car screeched to a halt right in front of us. Two burly, red-necked cops leaped out. They came rushing over to a feeble, gray-haired black man who had fallen to the sidewalk. The deputies grabbed the man, but not to help him back to his feet. They hurled him, head-first, like livestock, into the back of their cruiser.

He said nothing, at least nothing I could hear. And no one on the sidewalk stepped forward to intervene.

But I couldn't believe the cruelty of what I had just witnessed. I started crying. And with the naïve boldness that only an eight-year-old can muster, I went racing over to the patrol car and yanked at the arm of one of the deputies. At this point, he was still leaning through the open car door, pushing the man onto the floor in front of the back seat.

"Stop," I yelled. "Please, stop."

The deputy just shooed me away with the back of his hand. And my father rushed over and grabbed me, hustling me back to the Buick.

My father didn't try to tell me that everything was okay, or that the sheriff was just doing his job, or that I should have minded my own business. I'm sure he was as disturbed by the scene as I was. He, my mother, and I just got back into our car, with the tears still in my eyes. Silently, we drove south out of town.

That memory of Alabama was still quite fresh a week or so later when, on our return trip to New York, we made a two-day stop in Washington, D.C. I was, of course, thrilled to visit the nation's capital, to see the White House and the Congress and U.S. Supreme Court, not to mention all the museums and statues and parks. I was truly captivated—that is, until we visited St. Matthew's Cathedral, the Catholic equivalent of a national basilica. Again, I learned how seemingly good people are capable of doing evil.

At the rear of this great church, a tastefully roped-off area caught my eye. I could almost hear my father's heart drop when I asked him what it was for.

"For the Negro Catholics," he said with obvious discomfort.

That scene from Tuscaloosa came racing back into my mind, and tears started welling up. I was sick all over again. I don't know whether I was more confused or ashamed. But I certainly didn't understand how a church I knew I loved, a church I already knew I wanted to serve, could do such a terrible thing—could condone or even allow by its silence such an outrage to exist.

I was just eight years old that summer. But eight is plenty old enough to recognize something as painful as that.

The summer of 1932 was a very long time ago, but despite the passing years, I have never buried the hurt I felt on those two days. I'd like to think it made me a little more sensitive to the plight of the disadvantaged and to the essential role that the church must play as society's quintessential "change agent."

This is not such a complicated concept, and it's all laid out in the New Testament: We must comfort those who are needy, and we must confront those who are comfortable.

Too often, the church has done just the opposite, or has turned its eyes as others have done. Until we get this straight, how dare we say we walk in the footsteps of the Lord?

The purpose of religion is—and always has been—to change man's condition, to reconcile those who are adrift, to reconnect those who are cut off. This last one is especially important. So many people today need to be reconnected—vertically, with a loving Father, and horizontally, with loving peers. That, truly, is religion's job: reconnecting those who have been disconnected. Far too often, the leaders of my church and of others seem not to have learned this, or to have let it slip from their minds.

A road map is even included in the word *religion*, which comes from a Latin stem, *ligare* (to bind, like a ligament) and the prefix *re-* (back again).

Hence, *religion* or *religare* connotes binding back together, reconnecting, reconciling, restoring man who finds himself woefully adrift.

John Henry Newman, the British intellectual giant and convert who became a cardinal of the church, wrote brilliantly on the underlying dichotomy here: the way our divine institution, the church, is clothed in human frailty.

Men Not Angels, Ministers of the Gospel, Newman called his great treatise. It has always served as constant reminder to me personally to keep on track.

You can appreciate then how excited I was, on my very first visit to the Vatican, to discover the powerful imagery represented by Rome's sweeping boulevard, Via Reconciliazione, the Avenue of Reconciliation. It leads from the Tiber up to the outstretched arms of Bernini's colonnades, then across St. Peter's Square to the towering heights of the basilica's cupola—reconciling, or reconnecting, man with his caring family on Earth and with his Father in Heaven. What powerful imagery. I'd like to think it has strengthened the resolve of generations of churchmen to keep in mind our incredible mandate, that Heaven has been placed in hands of flesh and bone.

Drug addicts—especially, the young addicts—are the lepers of today.

We have our own convenient way of insulating adults, like ourselves, from the social condemnation. Doctors, lawyers, nurses, teachers, and business people who get hooked on drugs are classified as "occupationally impaired." Young people—caught in exactly the same behavior—are "criminal addicts."

That linguistic difference alone says a great deal about our world and about how quickly we are willing to write off our young.

When it comes to drug abuse, especially among the young, what we have heard from most of the religious community is a convenient, deafening silence.

That, and a trio of misreadings that almost guarantee their paltry efforts will come to naught. Sadly, they've chosen to take the comfortable way out. And this has meant a grave desertion of responsibility.

Misreading No. 1: *Drug addiction is fundamentally a conflict between good and evil—and, consequently, a conscious choice to sin or not to sin. Confession and repentance, therefore, are the churchly way out.*

Not long ago, one of the most powerful leaders of the American church climbed into his pulpit on Sunday morning and issued a resounding plea to drug addicts and others who have "fallen away" from the church:

"Repent!" he said. "Repent!" Such calls, I am afraid, are unlikely to do much about drug abuse.

These church leaders may feel terrific echoing the words of John the Baptist and following through on their sacerdotal mandate to recover sinners. Unfortunately, with young drug abusers, this is more self-serving than redemptive. And it pains those of us who are struggling daily to patch up the lives of the young.

You can't tell a youngster who has been victimized by sexual abuse or abandonment and who tries to block out the nightmare with drugs, "Repent!" You certainly cannot say "Repent!" to a youngster in the grip of cocaine or heroin addiction—and expect the call to be heard.

Life just doesn't work like that.

Heaven has a stake in the totality of life, both the human and the divine—and all of life's crises. Those of us in the church must always remember that. The "City of God" is inextricably woven into the "City of Man." Much hard work is left to be done. Saving souls includes saving lives. Far too often what we've been left with is just the kind of eyes-closed ignorance I saw at that cathedral in Washington all those years ago.

We can no longer afford to say, "Repent!" and then call it a day. Our problems are just too complex for that.

Misreading No. 2: *Drug addiction deserves no special attention or sympathy.* This is accepted rationale for doing nothing, and it has many proponents in the church. You know the idea: There's a whole range of painful afflictions out there—cancer, heart disease, muscular dystrophy, you name it—that deserve our attention and sympathy because innocent people are victimized. But in the case of addicts—well, their illness is self-inflicted and is something they could just as easily avoid. So let them swim in their own stew. Besides, if these kids weren't in trouble with drugs, they would be in trouble with something else.

I remember hearing just those words from the lips of a very distinguished and very religious business tycoon. It was interesting that this distinguished citizen, a good person and good friend, swiftly shifted gears when his own child ended up among the addicted.

The truth, of course, is that many of these so-called legitimate diseases contain a measure of self-infliction. Smoking, it seems to me and to most medical experts, contributes to cancer, heart disease, and stroke. Overeating, drinking to excess, and a lack of exercise all contribute to various ailments, some of them life threatening.

Sure, addiction has its willful elements. But many young addicts are throwaway kids who have suffered, beyond our wildest imagining, the horrors of physical abuse, sexual torment, or bleak abandonment, in an era when family life is on the ropes. They reach out to self-medicate. Simply blaming them falls far short of the moral accountability that I learned about in theology class.

Misreading No. 3: *We're already doing our part. We sponsor a couple of programs, after all.*

Why we help, as religious people, and how much we help: Those are not easy questions, even for the devout.

Essentially, the answer lies at the crossroads of what I call the "spiritual salvation needs" of the religious donor or Good Samaritan—pitted against the plight, both human and divine, of the cliffhanging needy one (in this case, the addict). This is the basic social challenge for any religious person. It merits serious reflection.

Every religion has a version of this mandate. "As long as you have done it unto one of these, you have done it to me" (the Christian mandate, recorded in the New Testament). "To save one life is enough to gain Heaven's reward" (the Jewish mandate, recorded in the Talmud).

This, at base, is the reason we reach out to feed the hungry, shelter the homeless, clothe the shivering and shelter the child. We do it not only because it is the right thing to do but because doing less would betray our own religious roots and jeopardize our own spiritual survival. So when we are stopped on the street, we pass on a quarter to the beggar, and he passes quickly out of our lives.

If you take a hard look at this, you might discover some tarnished religious motivations. He's gone, thank the Lord, and I didn't fail to properly acquit myself, spiritually. That was a close one!

But don't our responsibilities to the truly needy go deeper than that? Is that all that is meant by "resurrection"?

I may feel wonderful about giving the quarter or the warm coat or even the Thanksgiving dinner, and I may have advanced my own cause by buying "insurance" for Heaven's reward. But in this whole equation, where is the tragically desperate, needy person after I leave? Is he still on the street in his suffering? Is she still forced to peddle her wares in the shadows and in such agony? The fundamental issue for Christians and Jews and other believers ultimately focuses on that issue—the needy's resurrection versus the donor's salvation.

Put another way: Should I "give a fish for food for a day or teach the person how to fish for food for a lifetime." Admittedly, these are complicated issues for good people, even those prompted by splendid religious motivation. But somehow, I am certain, we are responsible for targeting our charitable actions toward the resurrection of the needy—not just toward our own spiritual gain—especially, when the two come into conflict.

That brings us to the addict and the alcoholic, those infantile, character-disordered people whom Daniel Casriel helped us understand. They are the emotional infants, rationalizing and fleeing the pain of their lives through chemicals and manipulating whomever they must to preserve their path to self-destruction. What does the church offer to them?

Religious people are conditioned to help. The addict or the alcoholic is quite aware of this and will swiftly channel these well-motivated energies into sympathetic intervention, which will buy time and some solid support for the journey down the road of slow death. *Mirabile dictu!* The religious benefactor has been positioned into the role of "enabler"—enabling the addict to continue his plunge.

In the past three or four decades, while working in parishes—those branch offices of the church—I am certain I was not the only priest who experienced a deluge of alcoholics and drug addicts at the rectory door.

At first, I did what priests are instructed to do. I called our human-services agency, Catholic Charities. It's a wonderful organization, energized in 1934 by a true visionary, Monsignor Robert Keegan, to respond in a structured, fine-tuned fashion to those in need.

For three decades after its founding, Catholic Charities chartered a truly remarkable record of achievement, especially among the needs of the young. The focus: orphaned and abandoned children.

Major institutions, incorporating the warmth and caring of home, were launched, and they carved an enviable record. In New York alone, almost two dozen of these big orphanages were opened, homes staffed by caring nuns. The most celebrated was Mount Loretto on Staten Island, overlooking Raritan Bay, which was founded by the legendary Father John Drumgoole and staffed by the splendid Sisters of St. Francis of Hastings. Sister Mary Reginald, a towering figure in my life, still labors there. The Blauvelt and Sparkill Dominicans defined their missionary commitment in the church by having wonderful orphanages in conjunction with their mother houses.

But by 1964, Catholic Charities suddenly found itself, three decades into its life, in the midst of a major social change. The orphaned or physically abandoned child was fast being replaced by a different profile of need: emotionally scarred, delinquent children. New needs call for new responses, and the time had come for a clinical retooling at Catholic Charities. The old responses— food, clothing, shelter, caring, and religious values—weren't enough anymore. The new kids already had homes and clothing and food. But still they were falling out of their families as a result of a new pattern of destructive parental behavior.

Unfortunately, Catholic Charities mostly dropped the ball.

Rather than abandon the traditional, now obsolete approaches at their child-caring institutions, or at least fine-tune them, Catholic Charities clung to yesteryear and continued its adherence to the classic social-work model.

A terrible tragedy followed.

The new breed of youngsters acted out to the horror of staff: smashing windows, setting fires to the buildings, assaulting the staff. Catholic Charities had no inkling of what to do. And it didn't take long for those two dozen wonderful institutions, launched with the vision of Monsignor Keegan, to shrink to two or three. These two or three will soon be gone also. And I am sure that the dedicated staff are content that they remained true to their Catholic social-work model, while the new breed of needy children remained beyond the rim of any saving graces whatsoever.

Along the way, Daytop offered to embark on a joint project with Catholic Charities in behavioral-modification treatment, which is precisely what we use successfully with the same deviant youngsters. The offer was turned down. I blame myself for failing to press on. Regardless, Catholic Charities has become a relic on the shelf of child care.

It was little wonder then that, when the subject of drugs came up in the parishes of New York in the 1950s and 1960s, the response from Catholic Charities more often than not was: "That's not our job! It's government's responsibility!" As if that were an answer to anything.

If the answer could not be found in the pages of the social workers' handbook, then the church didn't want responsibility. And the Catholic service agency was not alone in resisting this fundamental change. Both the Federation of Protestant Welfare Agencies and the Jewish Child Care Agency network stood by while the curtain fell on many of their child-care institutions.

What this history means is that, for organized religion, the topic of drug addiction has been a no-man's-land. "Stay far away from it." That's the message that has been transmitted to the religious and the laity. And it's left a gaping vacuum of concern. How else to explain the leading role Catholic parishes so often play in trying to keep drug-treatment centers out of their neighborhoods?

To me, nothing is sadder than this.

Daytop has felt the pain of thirty years of apathy and rejection on this front, beginning that first year back on Staten Island.

I recall, back in high school, how I marveled over the poet Francis Thompson's "The Hound of Heaven." God's love is boundless and stalks the steps of the most wayward prodigal. Another fan of the poem was the Jesuit Father John Magan, who worked with us at Daytop through the 1970s and 1980s, until Heaven called him home.

Father Magan researched the poem and discovered that Thompson was a drug addict and the poem actually was a saga of his own painful wandering, unable as he was to travel beyond Heaven's loving concern.

Heaven has been there most often in the constant concern of Rabbi Ron Sobel of Temple Emanu-El for the unfortunate of our town; in the great Reverend John Gensel of Manhattan's St. Peter's Lutheran Church in his ministry to the entertainment industry; in Jesuit Father Joe Toal's pounding the pavement of the drug-infested alleys of the South Bronx's Hunts Point area; in Father John Flynn's spelling out Christian compassion on the battle-scarred streets of Highbridge; in Father John Jenco of the Bronx's Bedford Park mobilizing the neighborhood to meet the drug threat; and in countless other ministries that would warm your heart as much as they do mine.

These are some of the notable standouts on this otherwise bleak landscape. The others are often young, devoted clergymen, of various faiths, who have come to the side of recovery. Yes, Damien continues to bring Heaven's loving concern to the lepers.

Still, sad to observe, those charged with leadership in the Christian community—the pastors, the vicars, the bishops, and the rest of them—have been notable mainly by their silence.

MYTHS, MYOPIA, AND MISCHIEF **17**

> *Whatever the form or constitution of government may be,*
> *it ought to have no other object than the general happiness.*
> *When, instead of this, it operates to create and increase*
> *wretchedness in any of the parts of society, it is on a wrong*
> *system, and reformation is necessary.*
>
> —Thomas Paine, *The Rights of Man*

Americans love easy answers. Deep down, most of us find ourselves prey to the quick fix. We're ready to believe even the most transparent charlatans, if their promises are grand enough and we don't have any better ideas of our own. Just think about how much time and money has been wasted over the years on miracle diets and sex-appeal toothpaste and get-rich-quick schemes.

We're like junkies in that way: we crave instant gratification.

The social consequences of this might not be so frightful when we're talking about, say, false baldness cures. What's really at stake there besides the vanity of a few middle-aged men? But when the easy-answer crowd begins hovering over the subject of drug use— watch out. The very lives of our young people are on the line.

If we are ever going to roll back the tide of drug abuse in America, first we must dispel a few seductive myths that have sidetracked our efforts for years.

These old canards get trotted out almost every time the topic turns to drugs. "Lock up the addicts!" someone will shout. "That'll solve the problem!"

"Seal the borders!"

"Execute the kingpins!"

Or, on the other side of the political spectrum: "Just legalize it!

People have a right to kill themselves if that's what they want to do!"

And what about the children? "Oh, yes, the children. Tell them to just say no!"

Confident-sounding answers, every one of them. And every one of them brutally simplistic, as well as fundamentally, provably wrong.

These simpleminded prescriptions and a few others like them make up what I call the Ten Crippling Myths of Drug Abuse. For decades now, we have been investing our hope in these myths. Every year or two, the nation wakes up and decides again that something must be done about drugs. But instead of giving serious thought to the question of what, we turn where we've been turning for years. We dust off one of the comfortable old myths and hope for the best. Almost always, the myth fails us—fails painfully, fails demonstrably, fails right out in the open. Yet when the next time comes around, we forget our disappointment. We ignore the pathetic results, and we invest another surge of optimism in one of these long-discredited myths.

The problem with most of them is that they ignore the basic cause of drug addiction, which is the crisis in the American family. Instead of confronting that sticky issue, the politicians, the law-enforcement officials, the think-tank media stars, and so many of the other widely trusted experts would rather pander. Their easy answers prove irresistible. So does their tough talk. And we keep throwing our hope and our dollars in the same unpromising directions we've been throwing them for years.

Like a nation of hard-core drug addicts, we cannot seem to stop ourselves.

Myth No. 1: *Since drug abuse is essentially a self-inflicted illness, the criminal law can be an effective deterrent—if the penalties are harsh enough.*

"I'll tell you how to solve the drug problem," someone will say, and not just reactionary hard-hats, either. "Lock 'em away forever. If that doesn't work, line 'em up against a wall and shoot a few of them. That'll make the rest of them think twice before messing around with drugs."

This "get tough" stuff is one of the most seductive myths in America's so-called war on drugs. The macho syllables create the impression that there is movement on the drug problem. We have spent billions, wasted decades, and packed the nation's prisons— all because of this mistaken belief.

The get-tough crowd has recently discovered the idea of military-style boot camps for arrested drug addicts. Discipline and hardship are heaped onto the addicts, as if that alone will cure anyone. In fact, the boot-camp idea is nothing new. It's been used for years in Singapore and Malaysia, with dismal results. Most of the addicts return to drugs the minute they hit after-care. Both those countries are now looking for new answers by experimenting with Daytop-style therapeutic communities.

Unfortunately, the threat of punishment is not nearly as potent a deterrent as people like to believe. The option of drug use is not so easily foreclosed. The nation's prisons are packed with inmates doing ten-, twenty-, and thirty-year sentences for drug-related crimes. Today, America holds a million of its citizens behind bars. And this hasn't made a dent in the supply of drugs on our streets.

The whole notion undercuts the reasons that young people choose to use drugs in the first place. Yes, there is an element of self-infliction here—just as there is with lung cancer, heart disease, and a whole range of other ailments. And yes, people should be held accountable for the things they choose to do.

But rarely is the decision to use drugs a product of some careful cost-benefit analysis. The prospective heroin junkie does not sit down and say, "Let me compare the pluses and minuses of a life on the needle." If that were the way life unfolded, no one would ever choose to take drugs, whatever the legal penalties might be.

People use drugs for lots of reasons: boredom, pain, risk, adventure, acceptance by their peers. "Getting tough" doesn't answer any of these. And it doesn't answer the underlying issue, which is the social crisis and the family crisis in America. Young people self-medicate as a means of blocking out their physical abandonment or their emotional pain. They use drugs as a balm for child abuse, sexual abuse, and a host of other ills. Jail cells simply reinforce all that loneliness and alienation and rejection, and they exacerbate the anger, frustration, and fear.

Myth No. 2: *If we can cut off the supply of crack (or high-grade heroin or methamphetamines or angel dust or whatever else happens to be the scare drug of the moment), things will get instantly better.*

We're always chasing after one "killer drug" or another. We almost never succeed in rooting it out. Eventually, fashions just change, and that drug gets replaced by another one—probably worse.

We've done this dance so many times the moves by now are almost predetermined: Articles appear in the papers about some horrific new street drug. Frequently, the stories are planted by the local narcotics cops, or by their state or federal counterparts. A few well-covered drug busts follow in short order, and public concern begins to rise. The law-enforcement officials say they are beginning to get on top of the latest scourge. But their efforts would be a whole lot more effective if the police budget were increased.

Frequently, the horror stories contain a measure of truth, even when the details are exaggerated. Whatever the drug of the moment, no doubt it can do awful things.

But all this law-enforcement showmanship doesn't add up to very much: a few high-profile busts, some self-congratulatory press conferences, a handful of bad guys marched off to jail, and a world that's barely changed at all.

And even if—miracle of miracles—the police somehow succeed in eliminating the supply of a particular dangerous drug, another one will appear on the scene right away. If history is any guide, the new one will be even worse.

Myth No. 3: *If we secure our borders and put pressure on the countries where the drugs come from, we can stop the crippling chemicals from ever reaching our streets.*

This is a pipe dream, and elementary school geography is only one of the reasons.

We share a border with Mexico of 1,933 miles. The Canadian-American border 3,987 miles. And don't forget the coastlines: 2,069 miles on the Atlantic Ocean, 7,623 miles on the Pacific and another 1,631 miles on the Gulf of Mexico. The country is simply too huge to build a fence around. When you factor in the millions of international visitors every year (legal and illegal), the megatons of cargo, and the who-knows-how-many parcels that go back and forth—well, you get the picture.

Many times a day, drugs and other contraband are seized at the borders. But the customs agents will be the first to tell you what a tiny fraction of the total ever falls into their net.

Every few years, some of our elected leaders start clamoring about the "unprotected borders." A "Caribbean Initiative" or some other bold-sounding program is announced. The usual press conferences are held. A few arrests are made. And the drug importers go quietly about their business, smuggling their foreign-grown poisons onto our shores. In fact, the drug pipeline flows more smoothly than it ever has. In the past decade alone, the supply of cocaine on the streets of America is up more than 200 percent.

This "seal the borders" talk is an extremely marketable myth, especially for politicians. It permits them to swagger around the drug issue, vowing to stand up to the deadly threat from abroad. And it allows the rest of us to blame "the foreigners" for a problem that is fundamentally our own. It's main-street America—not Lima, Bogotá, or La Paz—that is the engine driving our drug crisis.

In the end, this whole idea is doomed for the same reason that dooms other supply-oriented answers to the drug equation. It ignores the equation's more important half.

Supply and demand must be dealt with together. Drugs are not pushed on the American people by outsiders. They are brought into the country by our extraordinary level of demand. If Americans didn't buy the drugs, all those other countries would have no reason to export them. As long as there's such a lucrative market here, someone will find a way to serve it. Wouldn't it be a whole lot smarter to spend all that energy getting our kids off drugs?

Myth No. 4: *If we take the criminal penalties out of buying and selling drugs, the profit motive will disappear. Then, the drug merchants will have no reason to push their deadly wares and, eventually, the whole problem will evaporate.*

There are several things wrong with this idea, appealing though it may be. Most importantly, it misunderstands why young people use drugs in the first place. The reason is not pressure from unscrupulous dealers. It's that the users want what they believe the drugs have to give—risk and adventure, escape from reality, acceptance by their peers, a sense of belonging they had otherwise failed to achieve. Taking away the criminal penalties does not come close to answering any of that. It simply makes the drugs easier and less expensive to get.

At the same time, legalization brings with it some other thorny questions: Once we have publicly sanctioned the use of mind-numbing drugs, what do we say to the generation of young people who decide that, yes, they want to get high? Yes, they like to block out pain. Yes, they enjoy this sort of dysfunction. No, they don't mind the risks. What happens when these young drug users become nuclear technicians or police officers or airline pilots or train engineers? What happens when your own child is the one who is making this "choice"?

And what about the health dangers? We know that, over time, drug users build up tolerance to the chemicals. The more drugs they use, the more they need to kill the pain. Eventually, the doses reach lethal levels. What then? Are we comfortable just saying, "Good riddance"?

Some people argue that by taking the criminality out of the drug business, we also remove the allure of deviance—part of what draws young people to drugs. To some extent, this may be true. But the overall effect is likely to be something that no one wants: a more-open, more readily available pool of drugs and an even greater number of young people diving in.

Other countries have tried various versions of legalization. England conducted free-drug experiments back in the 1960s and abandoned the idea. So did Sweden and the Netherlands. In the United States, there is little reason to believe the results would be any different.

Myth No. 5: *Why muck around with complicated issues like the crisis in the American family? A big educational campaign, using newspapers and television and the rest of the mass media, can roll the drug problem back.*

Remember Nancy Reagan and her "Just Say No" campaign? That was a perfect example of Myth No. 5. So are those melodramatic TV commercials, like the one that shows an egg being fried: "This is your brain," the announcer intones. "This is your brain on drugs."

Big-budget media extravaganzas like those don't do any harm, I suppose—other than to divert people from more important efforts. And if they convince even a tiny number of people to think twice before taking drugs, so much the better.

But the sad reality is that most people learn about drugs not from the mass media but from their family and friends. The much touted power of the media is no match for the persuasiveness of drug-using classmates.

And these flashy ad campaigns do nothing at all for the veteran drug user. It's far too late for that, and the grip of drugs is too tight. All the razzle-dazzle is about as relevant to a heavy drug user as a

Pap smear is to a uterine cancer patient—or an antismoking ad to someone gasping with emphysema.

Any convincing should have been done a long time ago. What this requires is a counterforce a thousand times stronger than a TV ad.

One positive note: On this bleak horizon, by far the best prevention campaign is the one run by the Partnership for a Drug-Free America. The Partnership, which is funded by the private sector and headed by former Johnson & Johnson CEO Jim Burke, has carefully calibrated its mass media to reach what is really the only reachable audience—potential and casual users. The campaign's creators are to be commended for recognizing that real drug addicts are simply beyond the reach of such efforts. Using clear, confrontational messages, based on hard data and wrapped in the most convincing media packages, the Partnership has had noticeable impact on changing public attitudes. The public, I believe, has come to better grasp the reality surrounding the drug crisis. The prevention messages bang away at denial, leaving no place to hide. America owes an unpaid debt of gratitude to Burke and the Partnership.

Myth No. 6: *Okay, maybe the media isn't the answer. Then parents should teach their children to stay off drugs. Prevention, after all, is the real goal.*

Sure, prevention is important, and parents have a vital role to play. They should always try to set the best possible examples and encourage their children to stay away from drugs. Few forces are a bigger threat to a child's healthy upbringing than watching a mother or a father abuse drugs. Unfortunately, this is no longer such a rare event. The Woodstock generation are the parents of the 1990s, you know.

Where parents show their children constructive parental love, chances are the children will learn the vital lessons of self-discipline and responsibility. Such children are well on their way to real maturity. Rarely do such children desert so nourishing a family for drugs. This is prevention at its strongest point.

Having said that, however, let's not forget the other side of America's family life. Turmoil, physical or emotional abuse, lack of parental modeling, the drowning of children in permissiveness—these are the forces that create the walking-wounded child who is so vulnerable to negative peer influences. The families our children don't find at home, they build on the street. The day is then won by negative messages with social reinforcement. These children are beyond the reach of parental messages. They might hear the words, but they will never absorb the meaning. Parental-prevention efforts are much too late.

Figure that a typical addict, out there on Main Street America, will bring in three or four new recruits every month. Parents might think they have an influence over their own children. But the influence that the friends hold is far stronger. If those friends are pulling in a negative direction, all the at-home parent-child drug chats don't have much of a chance.

Myth No. 7: *Drug addicts are responsible for so much of the street crime in America, we really have no choice but to lock them up for long jail terms. This may not cure anyone's addiction. But at least it will protect the rest of us from the addict-criminals.*

It's true that serious drug addicts have a constant and almost insatiable need for money. And it is true also that addicts do some terrible things—rob, cheat, steal, manipulate, abuse—to get money for drugs. Obviously, society has a right to try to protect itself from this antisocial behavior.

But what we do is so clumsy that our efforts are bound to fail. Pass tougher laws. Impose stiffer sentences. Build more jail cells. That's about the extent of our repertoire. And then, we all act surprised when the problems keep getting worse.

We've been using the criminal law to fight drug addiction for many years now. It returned to high vogue during the get-tough Reagan years. It completely failed to reduce the number of drug users. New addicts were being minted on the street every hour, and many of the ones in jail were even finding ways to sustain their drug use behind bars.

What this has done is create a new number-one growth industry in America: prisons. We are now approaching one million Americans behind bars. One in four young black men is under the jurisdiction of the criminal-justice system. We shouldn't let ourselves forget what goes on in most of those prisons. They are expensive. They "reform" almost no one. They are universities that train people for larger crimes. The graduates come back onto the street, rougher and more desperate than they went in. It is not an exaggeration to say we are teaching these people how to destroy us.

Myth No. 8: *Addiction is irreversible. Trying to cure these people is nothing but a waste of time.*

We hear this sort of talk every time another big institution tries and fails to get a grip on the problems of drug addiction. The American landscape is littered with the programs and professions who gave up the fight in frustration. And to be fair, this is not an easy task.

But like many so-called experts, they found it difficult to admit their failure. Instead, a snappy phrase was invented: "Once an addict, always an addict." In other words, don't blame us experts if we fail.

It turns out, however, that the problem wasn't only the intractability of drug addiction, although dealing with addicts can be tremendously frustrating. The bigger problem was how these experts went about their work.

Just because they failed doesn't mean everyone will. The best proof of this is the phenomenal success that some drug-treatment programs have achieved. At Daytop alone, it's seventy-five thousand young people who, with a little help and a lot of work, have been able to turn around their lives.

We don't throw up our hands. We figure out what works. And not by any means are we the only people providing successful treatment. In the thirty years since Daytop was founded, hundreds of other programs around the world have taken up our model.

It isn't easy. It takes a huge commitment from the addicts and the staff. But it can work miracles. The best proof we have are all those former addicts walking around drug free. And as productive, responsible citizens, their taxes have repaid many times over the cost of treatment. Without that treatment, many of them would no doubt have continued to drain the public treasury as welfare recipients, prison inmates, or financial burdens of some other type.

Thankfully, they didn't believe the old slogan about "always an addict." Neither do we.

Myth No. 9: *The world is blessed with so many helping professions today—medicine, psychiatry, pharmacology, sociology, criminology, pedagogy, religion, to name just a few. Surely one of them must hold the key.*

We've spent most of the last century believing this. We bounced from one expert to another. We were sure that one of them had to hold the key.

The doctors tried to cure addiction. The psychiatrists took their turn, too. The sociologists and criminologists stepped forward—one with a blistering critique of the social order, the other with high walls and steel bars. The pharmacists mixed up promising potions. Students of the East even raised the hope of acupuncture cure. Christian fundamentalists swore Jesus was the only answer. Others put their faith in thirty-second TV spots.

Ever since America decided that drugs were a national problem, our nation has been putting its faith in one profession at a time. Not one of them has made much headway. The landscape of the drug-rehab business is littered with the debris of all their failed attempts.

If the last hundred years have taught us anything, they have taught us this: The whole human being needs healing. Taking care of one part is never enough. Thus, each of the helping professions has a role to play. Each one has special insights and tools to offer. No one of them can do it alone.

But when they work in concert—when the doctors and the psychiatrists and the social workers and the teachers and the ex-addicts join hands—amazing things can happen. People can be reborn.

Myth No. 10: *The American public is docile enough to accept these failures forever.*

This is the most prominent myth of all, and it has been a guiding principle in America's sputtering war on drugs.

But public patience, I believe, is finally wearing thin. People in this country are coming to the end of their collective rope. They are losing faith in the televised drug busts, the helicopters in Bolivia, the terror-drug-of-the-week, the saccharine Just-Say-No campaigns, the omnipresent urine specimens, the slamming of more and more cell doors—and all the rest of the high-priced theater that masquerades as our national policy against drugs.

For years, these theatrics have cast a mesmerizing spell at the ballot box and in the appropriation committees of Congress and the state legislatures. TV has played the barker to a gullible public. "Film at eleven!" the anchorman promises. And millions of us stare naïvely at the screen.

Well, people are finally beginning to realize what a huge failure all this hocus-pocus has been.

Their neighborhoods have been transformed into battle zones. There is no safety on the street—and not just in poor areas anymore. People no longer want to be massaged by all these dramatic weekend events. They are demanding action now. They are ready for a bona-fide movement against drugs.

We live in a push-button society, and like drug addicts we'd all prefer an instant response. That won't happen on a subject as complex as drug abuse. But we as a society must take a hard look at the reality that the problem is based in family life. We must therefore field a comprehensive response to the problems of the family itself.

It won't be quick. It won't be easy.

But we have so few choices. Most people, I believe, are more than ready to begin.

FROM BROOKLYN
TO BANGKOK 18

The more the movement spreads, the more individuals experience themselves as unique and choosing persons, deeply cared for by other unique persons—the more ways they will find to humanize our currently, dehumanizing forces... an avenue to personal fulfillment and growth.

—Carl Rogers, *Encounter Groups*

It was a warm April evening in 1980. Our brand-new Daytop-Italy Family Association had gathered in Piazza Cairoli in Rome. This was their fourth or fifth meeting together: a grand total of fourteen anxious moms and dads in one small room. What a far cry this was from the many thousands of family members who now show up each week for Daytop-style therapy groups all across Italy.

These first fourteen all had kids in our inaugural center at San Andrea in southwest Rome. And the parents, of course, were getting their own version of Daytop treatment. The meeting had just opened when a middle-aged man stood up and faced me. His name was Marcello, and his words had a high, emotional edge.

He explained that, each week, he traveled from his home in Anzio for the group meetings in Rome. This reminded him of something, he said, he wanted to tell the group. Back when he was a teenager, he stood near his home and watched as the American Fifth Army, led by General Mark Clark, landed on Anzio beach. He described the joy he had felt then and his gratitude to the Americans for lifting the occupation of Hitler's forces and ridding Italy of Mussolini's rule.

"You made us free again, you Americans," Marcello said, his voice now starting to quake. "And we shall never forget you."

As he went on, tears began rolling down his cheeks. "But that is nothing," he said, "compared with what you and Daytop are doing for our children. I don't know how we can ever thank you for that."

Wow.

That scene keeps popping up in my mind when I walk the streets of Manila, São Paulo, Tegucigalpa, Kuala Lumpur, or Beijing. There's more than enough family tragedy to go all around the world. Since the family remains the basic unit of all societies, Daytop's approach to family healing is readily translatable into any national situation and adaptable into any culture. Torrential storms may be breaking around the family, but still, the family remains the staple of every people on Earth.

Today, Daytop has brought its healing grace to forty-two countries around the world.

Who'd have ever thought it possible?

We certainly did not start out with any grand expectations about saving the world. Daytop began as a fundamentally local organization with fundamentally local aims.

This was clear from that very first press conference back in September 1963, called to announce the launching of Daytop Lodge (soon to become Daytop Village). The event was held in the office of Brooklyn District Attorney Edward Silver, right across the street from Brooklyn Supreme Court.

George Beldock, the presiding justice of the Supreme Court's Second Department, was on hand that day. So were Joe Shelly, the chief probation officer, and Alex Bassin, the researcher from the probation department, who oversaw the incubation of the Daytop plan. Several local politicians also came around for the announcement. One was Stanley Steingut, a Brooklyn legislator who went on to a powerful leadership position in the state assembly.

These were the best-known people in the room. This, of course, was eons before Daytop's successes brought the big-name celebrities and corporate titans around. Over the years, Daytop came to regard this small group of politicos and court officials as among our most valuable supporters and friends. We look back on them as towering figures, who made extraordinarily generous contributions to the cause.

But that day in 1963, I don't think a single one of them had any idea where this new organization would end up. No one could even dream about international alliances or world movements to combat the convulsions of drug abuse. No one, in fact, spoke about anything beyond a small group of drug-using probationers from Brooklyn and Staten Island, the district Shelly's office covered. If a handful of drug addicts could be saved—well, who could hope for more than that?

Today, Daytop's influence extends all the way from Brooklyn to Bangkok, from the rolling hills of Connecticut to the drug dens of South America, from China to Africa to the former Soviet Union and to many, many places in between.

Despite our early, local roots, we realized quite quickly that Daytop's approach to drug abuse had value far beyond our small corner of New York.

I remember vividly my first real hint of this. It came more than twenty years ago. Archer and Eva Tongue, the director and associate director of the International Council on Alcohol and Addictions in Lausanne, Switzerland, had asked me to represent the organization at the Council of Europe Meeting on Drug Addiction, which was being held in Strasbourg.

At the opening session, the president of the Council of Europe delivered a stirring address, jolting me to attention by her surprising reference: "And in the United States of America, we take special recognition of the American response to drug addiction, Daytop Village." I was stunned but pleased, to say the least. For the first time, I sensed the far-flung impact our young Staten Island effort was having around the world.

But the questions about Daytop's broadening mission went back even farther than that. One day in 1965, a joint committee of the United States Congress had come to Daytop Staten Island to conduct a public hearing on what might be done about drug abuse.

The hearing went along as all hearings do. The various experts trotted out the usual "answers." Government witnesses were droning on. Finally, one of the members of the committee decided to ask some questions of the Daytop residents who had been sitting quietly in the meeting room.

"What would you think if America legalized drugs, took all the criminal penalties out?" the congressman asked one resident, a young man in his twenties who happened to be the nephew of a well-known state judge.

The legalization issue has been floating in and out of the public debate for many, many years. We actually did have legal drugs once. Remember those nineteenth-century opium addicts and their trips to the candy store? Still, we keep turning to the old canards like this. Bizarre, isn't it?

In any event, the congressman asked the legalization question, and this young resident stood up and spoke.

"I have a real problem with that," he said, looking the congressman in the eye. "What you're telling me is that you're thinking about licensing death for the young people of America. Is that what America is about?"

The congressman didn't say anything, at least not right away. But the words of this young resident seemed to hang over the room, even as other members of the committee asked questions of other residents. Later, several of the congressmen came up to say how impressed they had been with the candor of the young people who had spoken.

Then, the congressman who asked the legalization question walked over and introduced himself. He didn't sound at all offended by the young resident's riposte. "Father," he said, "I have to tell you how encouraging this place is, what a phenomenal achievement you have on your hands. Too bad it's just a drop in the ocean. The drug problem is just so huge. Even with a great program like Daytop, you must feel hopelessly overwhelmed sometimes."

My face must have fallen a little at that last comment because the congressman quickly apologized. This wasn't exactly how we saw our work, as hopelessly overwhelming. But despite the crude analogy, the congressman was right, in a sense, with his drop-in-the-ocean remark.

The problems caused by drugs are gigantic. They are spread liberally around the world. And back then at least Daytop had barely begun to respond.

"New York is the number-one impact area for drugs in America," I told the congressman. "But you're right about one thing. The problem is everywhere. We're going to have to figure how to reach some of those other people. But we can't allow ourselves to dilute the work we are able to do right here."

And over the years since that conversation, that's the careful path we've walked.

We've expanded, dramatically, in our own backyard. That amazing total keeps coming back to mind: Daytop New York has returned more than seventy-five thousand addicts to society, where the vast majority of them are living useful, productive lives. And the Daytop Family Association has reached almost as many families, helping to heal them as well.

We've gone from that one house on Staten Island, with a capacity of just twenty-five residents, to eighteen facilities, treating thousands of clients at any one time. We have a myriad of ancillary programs we never had before—the Mini-versity, Daytop C.A.R.E.S., the Promethean training center, the special groups for pregnant addicts and addicts who have AIDS. The list goes on and on.

But these New York–based programs are by no means the extent of Daytop's reach. Today, more than 3 million people are involved worldwide in what has become the Daytop movement. That one drop of water the congressman spoke about has grown into an ocean of its own.

Despite the strictly local ambitions at the time of Daytop's birth, the subject of expansion arose almost from day one. And not just expansion of our own program in New York.

We were soon getting numerous inquiries from cities and towns across America. People had heard or read about the things that were happening at Daytop, that addicts were successfully leaving their drug use behind. Word of Daytop's achievement spread extremely fast.

"Something very promising is going on there in New York," these people would tell us. "We'd like to have it here in Chicago"—or Philadelphia, or Connecticut, or any one of the countless other places we heard from.

This was flattering, of course. But it forced us to do some serious soul-searching early in our history about what the Daytop organization was going to be.

Our board of directors, which numbered only eight people, made a hard decision—but one that I believe turned out to be extremely wise. Our home turf, the board members recognized, had the most severe drug problem anywhere in the country, perhaps anywhere in the world. Trying to fight drugs in New York was likely to remain a challenge of tremendous complexity and size. Daytop should not, therefore, begin opening branch offices all over the map or taking other steps that would dilute our energies from the huge mission we already had. So the Daytop organization, the board decided, would confine itself to New York.

But that wasn't the extent of our answer.

We were still quite concerned about the kids in Chicago, Philadelphia, Connecticut, and all those other places. So we needed to come up with a way to keep our energies focused where they belonged, while at the same time sharing this life-saving knowledge that we had.

So this is what we told those people who were serious about facing the problem head-on:

"We have our hands full in New York. It would be a mistake—a big mistake—for us to begin running little Daytops all over the place. But we'd be happy to show you how to do it. We can teach you how to run a similar program on your own. And the Daytop Training Institute at Swan Lake was born in response to that need.

"We'll train your people in our methods. We'd be happy to lend you a couple of our staff members—maybe even a few residents—to get you on your feet. Our board will show your board what to do.

"But we want to emphasize, you must take responsibility for yourselves. Your problem is your problem, Chicago," or Philadelphia or Connecticut or wherever. "It's not New York's problem. You are the ones who are going to have to solve it. At Daytop, we teach each individual to take responsibility for his or her own life. We want you to take responsibility for your local drug problem.

"Also, if you start your own program, it should have its own name—something with some local flavor to go along with the universal goals. In the end, you will have to be responsible for yourselves."

And that's how it's been.

Over the years, many towns and cities in America have taken us up on that offer. So have many countries around the world. Leaders of these nascent efforts have been coming to visit us in New York. We've sent staff and residents back home with them and helped to create Daytop-styled programs of their own.

The result of these efforts is truly heartwarming. Today, second-generation Daytops have been established, with our hands-on guidance, in ninety-one American cities and towns and thirty-two countries around the world. Not every one of them has succeeded. But in the vast majority of cases, the local people have done fantastically well, establishing programs, raising money, taking over the training of their staff members, creating countless miracles of their own.

Many of those programs have gone on to inspire others. So we have hundreds of children and grandchildren out there, Daytop-inspired and many of them Daytop-trained.

This is the way our movement spread, and we are proud to have been the first to find the way to make it happen. It is one of the things that marked the difference between Daytop and our own forebears at Synanon.

Chuck Dederich had a longstanding interest in the expansion of Synanon. But his efforts in this regard were ultimately stymied by his insistence on running everything himself. He did succeed in opening several Synanon outposts, which were essentially franchises, micro-managed from the California headquarters. They blossomed briefly, but none of them lasted very long. They didn't have the flexibility and the local relationships that are so vital to a program's long-term success. They were hobbled, as well, by the intensifying madness at the home office.

We're still following the other path, constructing a gigantic movement out of these disparate local efforts. And so today, there's Gateway House in Chicago, Gaudenzia House in Philadelphia, Phoenix House in New York, Marathon House in Providence, the Village South in Miami, and on and on and on. Every one of them is taking the lessons they learned from Daytop and putting them to work for their own young people.

Before we knew it, a huge extended family was growing up. We were not carbon copies of each other, and we all faced special challenges of our own. But it was becoming increasingly clear how much we had to share with each other—first and foremost our fundamental belief in the self-help, drug-free approach to healing the entire person.

A similar process unfolded on the international front.

The U.S. State Department, in recognition of Daytop's obvious successes, has for years been referring officials from other countries to us. This came to be such a common occurrence we eventually set up a special branch of the organization to deal with these inquiries: Daytop International, under Executive Director Gerald Jeremiah.

We have provided technical guidance to so many countries around the world, it is impossible to remember them all.

I recall one early group of international visitors from Montreal, Canada, who appeared on our doorstep one day in 1970. The delegation was led by the members of the Howlett family, an old and civic-minded Montreal clan. They had grown very much concerned, they told us, about the drugs that seemed to be infecting their city's young.

They asked the usual question: Could they have a Daytop in Montreal? We explained to them that our board wouldn't permit that, but that we were concerned about the young people of Canada and we would show them how to set up a parallel organization of their own.

We sent them up to our adolescent center in Millbrook. They came back to the city almost speechless. We arranged for their new staff to come down and spend some time at Daytop. We sent a couple of our more experienced staff members up to Canada to guide them through the birthing process.

The result was Le Portage, Canada's first therapeutic-community program for drug addicts. It sprung to life and has been a beacon for the young people of Canada since 1971.

That was just the beginning. Similar things kept happening all over the world. It was only natural, therefore, for us to think about establishing some kind of formal structure to help promote these shared ideals, uniting therapeutic communities across the United States and, increasingly, in other parts of the world.

This happened in 1975, on the banks of the Chao Phraya in Bangkok, Thailand. The leaders of many of the most important therapeutic communities had gathered there as part of a conference of the International Council on Alcohol and Addictions.

Several therapeutic-community leaders had played important roles in the International Council. But they were growing more and more disenchanted with the traditional, medical approach that had held sway in the organization for so many years. Most of the council's members, we felt, were still falling into that old trap of focusing treatment on the drug—not the user—with all the usual failed results.

It was out of that feeling of frustration that the World Federation of Therapeutic Communities was born. We decided we could and should band together and stage international conferences of our own. We had some exciting things to talk about, after all, and a growing roster of professionals who were interested in our approach.

We held our first solo conference the following year in Sweden. The most important leaders of this growing movement traveled from five continents to be there. The event, everyone agreed, was a smashing success. The only complaint I heard was: Why hadn't we done this a long time ago? These world conferences have been staged in one country or another every year since: Canada, Italy, the Netherlands, the United States, the Philippines, Greece, with future conferences to be held in Malaysia (1993), Hungary (1994), and China (1995).

At the world conference in New York in 1979, a formal charter and a set of bylaws were drawn up. They were officially adopted the following year when we met in the Netherlands.

Despite the creation of our own group, we didn't abandon the old-line International Council, which has its headquarters in Lausanne, Switzerland. We continued as a distinct section of the council—one of its most active, incidentally. We believe we have a continuing responsibility to spread the lessons we have learned, even to our most uninterested colleagues. So we have pressed on in that effort, even when it sometimes seems to bog down.

As the World Federation's name implies, the Daytop movement has never been hemmed in by international borders. What we do can be applied anywhere, and we recognized this from our earliest days.

Probably the most exciting work anywhere is what's been going on in Italy. We held the world conference there in 1978, under the leadership of Don Mario Picchi. It was an awe-inspiring conference, as our meetings in Rome often are, with the appearances of a pope, a president, and the city's mayor.

Out of that conference came an anguished plea on the part of our Roman hosts to help them establish a therapeutic community for the young people of Italy. A few months later, on February 1, 1979, we sent over our first director, Richard Falzone. He opened a small center in southeast Rome in a tiny building that was loaned to us by the Belgian Sisters. It had room for fourteen young addict-residents, and two staff members in training.

Falzone's efforts in Rome were later supplemented with twelve other Daytop American staff, who took positions in the capital city and also at the centers that soon opened in Florence, Verona, and in other parts of Italy.

Various facilities have been placed at our disposal. None of them, however, is more wonderful than the training center we have helped set up at the House of the Sun, Casa de Sole, right across from the Pope's residence at Castel Gandolfo. It has proven to be an extraordinary boon.

We sent Anthony Gelormino from New York to get the training center up and running. One thousand Italian staff members have already been trained there. They now have moved into positions at 150 separate facilities in thirty-six towns and cities across Italy. Already, they have engaged ten thousand of the country's young people in recovery—and twice the number of parents in weekly therapy groups. It's almost like a revolution has occurred on the Italian peninsula. It is one of the brightest lights in our whole World Federation. And do you know what the best part is? The Italians are now running the whole thing without us.

All through the late 1970s and 1980s, the movement continued to spread. Sometimes it was to places quite like the United States. Other times, it was to places as different as can be.

We helped set up a successful program in Dublin. We sent staff to Sweden and helped set up a program there. Today, there are centers in five Swedish cities. And the Swedes have just jumped across the border to Norway, where a program will open soon. Again, it's the children begetting children of their own.

One of the highlights on the European continent is the tremendous Munich-based Daytop treatment network, which now has thirty-two centers all over Germany. Ulrich Osterhues, the director there, has turned Germany into a beachhead of hope.

Phoenix House, the stellar program in England, is another Daytop grandchild. Phoenix House New York grew out of Daytop Staten Island, and it was their people who helped England set up a program of its own. These influences are readily apparent by the presence of the Daytop philosophy posted at the door of the London Phoenix House.

The movement has spread in similar ways through the British Isles, throughout Scandinavia, to much of Eastern Europe and into the territory that was the Soviet Union.

The situation in the Netherlands was special. One of the most socially conscious parts of the world, the treatment community there never lacked interest or energy. But for too long, their good intentions were focused in exactly the wrong place.

In the early 1970s, the Jellinek Clinic in Amsterdam was being hailed across the world as a leader in the professional treatment of addictions to alcohol and drugs. But like many such clinics, it limped along with pathetic results. Huge amounts of money were spent and very few addicts were succeeding in changing their lives.

The Netherlands had little to feel encouraged about on this front until ten years ago. That's when the country's first therapeutic community, Emiliehoeve, was installed in The Hague. The usual positive results were achieved quickly there. And in a peculiar twist, the man who had founded Emiliehoeve, Dr. Martien Kooyman, then took the reins of the Jellenik Center and replaced the failed medical model with the therapeutic community.

Now we have a number of therapeutic communities across the Netherlands—led by Emiliehoeve in The Hague, in Hoogholen, and in other areas of the Netherlands. In Belgium, next door, there are now programs in Ghent and Bruges. And we are very pleased that both Hungary and the former Yugoslavia have responded dramatically to a growing youth drug crisis and have welcomed therapeutic-community training.

The particulars are different from culture to culture, but the model remains much the same.

In Greece, under the leadership of Dr. Phoebus Zaphirides, the results are already promising. A new program, called Kethea, has several centers in Athens and others in Thessaloniki.

In Israel, under the indomitable Abie Nathan, we will soon complete the largest therapeutic community in the Mideast, being built in the Negev. Initial training will be provided by Daytop International.

In all these places, we take advantage as much as possible of the local leadership: church, civic, or government groups—anyone really, whose heart and energies seem to be in the right place.

In Egypt, for instance, this has meant working with the Coptic Church. The very dedicated Bishop Serapian has gotten tremendously involved. We have sent over staff from Daytop International. He's done everything imaginable to smooth the way.

The focus in all these countries is for the local leaders to take the basic theories and apply them flexibly to the indigenous culture. This approach starts with the program's name and goes all the way through to the execution. The Daytop-inspired programs that have grown in Oceania—Australia, New Zealand, New Guinea, and the surrounding islands of the Polynesian and Micronesian chain—have done an especially admirable job. The Odyssey House program in New York, itself trained by Daytop staff, has led the charge in Australia and New Zealand, without running roughshod over local sensibilities. Ian Permezel of Melbourne's McCann Foundation has provided major impetus for the success of the Therapeutic Movement in that region. As my first vice-president of the World Federation of Therapeutic Communities, he has brought to the rest of the world his remarkable energies for saving young lives and is truly one of "Heaven's People." We are involved directly in the incubation of the therapeutic community in Papua, New Guinea, a program that will respect local attitudes and customs yet will still follow the basic precepts of honesty, confrontation, and Daytop's other fundamental themes. The leader there is Father Bill Liebert.

Latin America has not been without concern and movement.

In 1980, I visited our colleague agency, FUCABEM, in Brazil's resort city of Florianapolis, 300 miles south of Rio on the Atlantic. I saw the powerful, caring message of recovery unfold there in the lives of twenty-six thousand youngsters, from babies in bassinets to teenagers, all abandoned by their impoverished families in *favellas* of Rio, São Paulo, and Recife. A horrible reality to behold— but equally consoling to witness the caring hearts of the FUCABEM staff. Harold Rahm, a dynamic Jesuit and the "Father Flanagan of Brazil," has worked miracles on his *ranchos*, the therapeutic communities in Brazil, as has Lilia Catao in Rio.

Throughout Latin America, the drug problems speak in voices of dire poverty, with echoes of abandonment, fear, and violence. Marco Fidel Lopez Fernandez, a dedicated Franciscan, has "borne the burden of the day's heat" in pushing treatment sanctuaries in Bogotá, Medellín, and Cali in Colombia, a nation positively awash in cocaine. Patricia Ackerman is doing similar work in Bolivia's La Paz, where old-fashioned neglect is swallowing the young. In Argentina, Carlos Rossi, Carlos Novelli, and Daniel Campagna carry our banners of hope and recovery.

Our programs are rarer in Central America. But Felician Napoli, another Franciscan, is striking a spark on behalf of the preteen street kids of Tegucigalpa, Honduras, where glue sniffing has spread like an epidemic.

Asia is a complex and exciting story of its own.

In 1972, Daytop trained a cadre from Manila in the Philippines and brought them back the following year for retraining. Out of that came a program called DARE, which became the first therapeutic community in the South China Sea. The Philippine program grew steadily, approaching a population of a thousand residents in a very short time. The leaders there did exactly as we had hoped they would and began to show neighboring countries how to confront their own drug problems.

It's the old therapeutic-community axiom at work, the one that's up on the wall at every Daytop center: *You can't keep it unless you give it away.* The Malaysian program, in Ipoh, to the west of the Philippines, is called Pusat Pertolongan, The Helping Center. It is a child of DARE. The current director of Daytop International is the former assistant director of the Pusat program.

In turn, the Philippine program, DARE, was also instrumental in assisting Thailand in the establishment of the Rebirth Center in Ratchaburi, about an hour and a half outside Bangkok. We are currently working, via Daytop International, with Thailand's Narcotic Control Board and with the National Council of Social Welfare to establish sister programs in the most highly impacted areas of the country, such as Bangkok City, where we already conduct the Re-entry phase. There is also serious talk about the therapeutic community being organized in the area surrounding the port of Pattaya.

We have been met with open arms in Thailand by Bishop Thienchai and Cardinal Michai. I have no doubts that the movement's future there is bright. In neighboring Burma, we have come less far. In 1989, we trained three health leaders from the Burmese capital of Rangoon. They are back in their country now. We look forward to the beginnings of the movement there through their leadership.

Elsewhere in Asia, we have promising ventures in Sri Lanka, under the direction of Father Fernando; in Guam, under Father

David Quitaga; and in India, where the multicenter Seva Dhan program is based. It was founded originally by Russell Pinto, a truly committed therapeutic-community leader. We have seen some early momentum in Nepal and Indonesia.

In June 1990, at the invitation of the Ministry of Health in the People's Republic of China, we visited the health authorities in Beijing. Then, we traveled about two and a half hours by air into southeast China to Yunnan Province and its capital, Kunming. This is a very scenic region, bordering Tibet, Laos, Burma, and Vietnam in the valley of the Himalayas. But it is also a major international drug corridor, where opium comes down from Laos and is converted into heroin in Burmese labs.

Before setting out for Kunming, we whetted our curiosity by visiting Tiananmen Square, a few blocks from our hotel. It was a Sunday, a holiday, and the square was jammed with families. Just three months earlier, that brave boy had stood up to the tanks and thousands of other young people had battled beneath a makeshift Lady of Freedom.

The square is huge, perhaps as large as a half dozen football fields. The people there ran up to us. They seemed so relieved to see Westerners. Though a unit of soldiers jogged across the square every few minutes, their martial chants reminding everyone that "Big Brother" was nearby, the Chinese people were extraordinarily friendly and their children bathed in smiles. I just prayed for their future on that spot of martyrdom.

We got a warm welcome from Dr. Zuoning Jiang, a highly respected Beijing physician who is the director of the drug dependence unit at An Ding, the "Bellevue of Beijing." He remains a driving force behind the movement to bring Daytop to China. Luckily for us, his great enthusiasm is shared by the deputy minister of health, his health counterpart in Yunnan Province and the chief of the provincial drug dependence unit. Despite China's continuing political problems, I am confident that the drug-treatment movement has a bright future there.

In our tours of their facilities, we learned, interestingly, that the training of Chinese psychiatrists begins and ends with Pavlov. Not a very encouraging thought, is it? We also learned what low esteem acupuncture is held in as a method of drug treatment. It does help with the pangs of drug withdrawal, the Chinese believe. But they have found the approach to have no impact at all on recovery or on rebuilding an addict's life.

This last discovery brought a smile to my face. The day we left New York, the city health department had announced the opening of six publicly funded acupuncture clinics to cure drug addiction. Perhaps they should have checked first with the Chinese.

Once we got out to Yunnan, we were shocked to discover the size of the population of intravenous heroin users: 460,000 young people. We visited hundreds of them. They are beautiful, not so different from our own young people. Sadly, these Chinese addicts are self-medicating for the same reasons that our young people self-medicate: they want to block out the pain of their lives, caused and exacerbated by dysfunctional families. We spent hours chatting with these addicts. They are crying for help.

Along with the addiction problem, AIDS is now showing up there for the first time. Eight hundred and ten cases have already been counted. Surely, that is just the beginning of the epidemic among the province's needle-using young.

Soon, we will open twin centers in Yunnan Province—a treatment center and a staff-training center. A second phase of our attention will draw us to sprawling Canton. We are happy to begin our activities in China far from Beijing, which we found extraordinarily political and still very much in the shadow of the Tiananmen Square massacre. It will be wonderful to be able to include the world's most populous country in our international movement.

We are very concerned about Africa and have been for some while. Fifteen years ago, there was a therapeutic community in Capetown, trained by Daytop Germany. But the South African government insisted that we follow their onerous practice of apartheid. We told them we could not. They invited us to leave and we did.

Things there may finally be loosening up. New interest is being expressed and we are eager to find a way to return—on a racially integrated basis, of course. If this works out, the South African effort would join other nascent moves on the African continent, from the Ivory Coast, Mali, Kenya, and Nigeria. We are programming right now to respond to requests from them.

That, I believe, just about covers the world.

There are still some dry patches out there. But the ocean of hope has grown quite wide.

What began with a dream—a very local dream, in a district attorney's office in New York City and at a single house on Staten Island—is now a world movement of major proportions. It is recognized by the United Nations, as well as by the Council of Europe, the U.S. State Department, and a host of international agencies.

And the size of that one drop of water—3 million and counting—is still growing at a rate of 10 percent a year. Not bad, considering where we started out.

THEY DARED TO CARE 19

Encourage one another and build one another up.

—St. Paul's Epistle, *Thessalonians 5:11*

Teach and admonish one another.

—St. Paul's Epistle, *Colossians 3:16*

In this battle that we've been fighting over the past thirty years, we have had ample reason to become discouraged.

There's the shockingly high rate of mortality among America's young, her children, her future. There's the grave lack of national will to overcome the one problem that is claiming most of those lives. There's the maddening lack of leadership from the people who are charged with leading us. There's the deluge of government funding for the tired old approaches—and the shrugged shoulders for the answers that are proven to work.

The late Harry Sholl, who founded Chicago's Gateway House, used to shake his head in wonder and say with a smile: "This is the only war in America to be fought with nothing but words." Sadly, Harry knew what he was talking about. No one can work in this field for any length of time without occasionally being overrun by feelings of outrage and shame.

This is why we so treasure the individual heroes who have been there for us.

Their number isn't all that large. But many of them are people who have attained a certain position in society, who are comfortable, who could certainly afford to look the other way. Yet they are still moved by a genuine concern for the ones who need them most.

They are, as we say at Daytop, the ones who dare to care.

In the years since our founding, some extraordinary people stood by us when the pressure was greatest. They helped spread our message when no one wanted to hear it. They had advice when advice is what we needed most. They had encouragement when we were beginning to feel despair. They went out and leaned on their friends for money when our cupboards grew desperately bare.

These are people from the worlds of government and politics, religion and business, entertainment and sports. They differed from each other in countless ways. But all of them have had a few things in common. They cared for the kids. They cared for the future. They cared because caring was the right thing to do.

Our hats off to them.

And at the top of this Blue Ribbon Honor Roll are the men and women who have served on the Daytop Board of Governors and the Board of Trustees. Drawn from the ranks of key community leaders, they have given of themselves, day in and day out for three decades now, making sure we stayed our vital course. Seventy-five thousand young people stand in their debt.

But these shining lights go all the way back to our earliest days on Staten Island. Even at that time of great fear and hostility, a few brave people stood tall. They supported us publicly and carried our cause into what was often hostile territory, sometimes at real risk to themselves. And they did it for one reason alone: they believed in what we were trying to do.

I can't even remember some of their names. But they showed up at our house on frigid evenings, with food and warm clothing. I remember one couple coming by the day before Thanksgiving, with a giant cooked turkey and enough side dishes to ensure that everyone in the house would get seconds or thirds. Others appeared with donations to help with the fuel bill.

Many of these people were recruited by Pearce O'Callaghan and

Ruth Hagemann, two very caring community leaders on Staten Island. Pearce and Ruth were not scared of bucking public opinion and joining our fight.

There were a few young priests who also stood by us in those days. They had been touched by drug problems in their own communities and had come swiftly to our side. Fathers Pete Finn and Larry O'Connor were models of religion's social commitment.

And there was Monsignor Henry Vier, a splendid and highly respected Staten Island figure who ran the Catholic orphanage of Mount Loretto. Monsignor Vier's orphanage was right down the road from the Daytop house, and he might well have joined our raucous opponents.

Instead, he warmed us with encouragement and a genuine priestly concern, and he never tired of arguing our cause. He believed that the future of many young lives was at stake. Everyone on Staten Island knew this gentle, undaunted priest. In my view, he ranks among the giants of our world.

The monsignor showed the same kind of loving concern that, years later, Pope John Paul II would show to Daytop.

You wouldn't expect such a personal touch from a man in so lofty a position, weighed down as he must be by the countless issues competing for his time. But this pope has spent many, many hours at our centers in Rome and at our training facility at Castel Gandolfo. His energies have been directed toward raising the spirits of our residents, while focusing the attention of Italy, the church, and the world.

On one of his very first visits to Castel Gandolfo, in 1980, he spoke to the young people in eloquent terms about how important they were in the worldwide battle against drugs.

"If we have to conquer the major threat of drugs, we have to have some proof of the possibility of winning," he said. "If we have the certainty that we can win, the certainty proved by you people—the people who have won—then we can face the threat with great hope. You young people—who have won—serve as witnesses of hope of the victory that is possible. You provide, also, for society, which is so anxious about the problem of drugs. You provide them with an incentive to wage the battle, to draw upon all its strength, all its goodwill.

"It is worthwhile because victory is possible. You are the winners. You must convince young people around the world that it is possible to win."

Pope John Paul II has returned to our Italian affiliate frequently since then. And we have sent delegations of young people from Daytop America to visit with him. It was on one of those visits that he explained to our kids why they have touched him so much.

"You are the only ones asking the basic questions of life," he told them. " 'Why were we born? What are we doing here? What's the purpose of this journey called life? What's its meaning?'

"Very few people are asking these questions. They must be asked, and they must be answered. I salute you for seeking those answers and asking those important questions."

In Italy, there is no better patron to have than the pope. And the entire hierarchy of the Italian church seems to have heard his message loud and clear. This is one of the main reasons that Italy's drug problem is being dealt with in such a serious way.

I must say that this pope's predecessor, Pope John Paul I, was another shining light.

Before rising to the papacy, he was cardinal archbishop of Venice. Cardinal Luciano, as he was called back then, was a man known for his keen social conscience. One day, a Father Angelo requested a meeting with him at the chancery to discuss a touchy situation he had on his hands.

"Just when our work with the young addicts is finally going so well," the priest explained, after settling onto the cardinal's couch, "we have this to deal with." *This* was the police. "They are putting extreme pressure on us," Father Angelo said. It seemed that, under Italian law, anyone who knew about a drug addict was required to report that person to the authorities, so he or she could be arrested.

"They want me to turn in my own kids," Father Angelo said. "I can't stand the thought of doing that. We have developed a trust. And if we started calling the police, how many more addicts do you think would show up at our door?"

The cardinal paused for a second. Then he answered the priest. "Keep on doing what you're doing," he said. "You continue your work. That's where Jesus would be! I will go around to the parishes and get the people's support."

The pope told that story to Father Mario and me the first time we met him, shortly after his brief papacy began. But as he came to the end of the story, the pope's eyes began welling up with tears.

"I came to Rome three days later," he told us. "That's when they elected me pope. And poor Don Angelo—Father Angelo—is all alone now in Venice. I worry about him. I pray for him. Would you be able to go up there and see him? Give him whatever help he needs."

Then he switched into the third person, a manner of speaking that somehow never sounds pretentious coming from the head of the church. "It would greatly relieve the pope if you would do that," he said.

We got in a car that afternoon and drove straight off to Venice.

When I think back on all the wonderful experiences we have had in Rome, I become dumbfounded by the comparatively cold shoulder our cause has been shown by the American church.

True, there are hundreds of individual priests, nuns, and brothers out there who have done great work with drug addicts and with the families these addicts threaten to destroy. But when it comes time for the church's leadership to show its commitment, the hierarchy has mostly chosen not to get involved. This is in glaring contrast to the pope's open arms.

Over the past two decades, the American bishops have weighed in with formal statements on social issues of almost every stripe: welfare reform, the Middle East, Mexican workers, torture in Brazil, racism in South Africa, Nicaragua, Chile, Cuba, Panama, unemployment, the death penalty, American Indians, Southeast Asian boat refugees, El Salvador, Marxist Communism, the Polish church, AIDS, birth control, and many, many more.

But until November of 1990, the bishops never got around to addressing the central issue of drugs, this thing that has been gnawing away at the core of family life for such a long time. That month, for the first time in history, they finally sandwiched in a brief commentary on America's drug problem, among discussions of priestly formation, the war in Kuwait and the slaying of those Jesuit martyrs in El Salvador. Even our secular politicians have often done better than that.

Among our earliest friends in politics was the late Senator Thomas Dodd of Connecticut, whose son Christopher currently represents that state in the Senate. The elder Dodd was the one who rose on the Senate floor, wide-eyed about the remarkable program in Santa Monica, where drug addicts were recapturing their lives.

That was in 1960. Dodd stayed interested in the issue. In the years since, we've been lucky enough to encounter various other Tom Dodds—people entrusted with leadership who have stepped forward to be counted at the side of our tragic youngsters.

There is no question that Daytop has benefited immensely from its presence in New York State. The men who have led the state in that time have, without exception, all stood by us.

Perhaps Malcolm Wilson, who served as lieutenant governor and then governor during our formative years, deserves special credit for focusing state government on the drug problem and on Daytop's value to kids in New York. But the other three—Nelson Rockefeller, Hugh Carey, and Mario Cuomo—shared the same unique grasp of the problem and the commitment to do something about it. They all saw in Daytop a well-tested response that offered hope and did so at reasonable cost.

New York State Senator John Marchi was another one who remained a touching figure of great compassion and courage. He has been a breath of fresh air to all of us in the field, sometimes at considerable cost to himself.

Marchi represents Staten Island, where many of the early battles over Daytop were fought. From the beginning, Marchi showed himself to be a man of supreme integrity, dedicated to those qualities that should be a touchstone for everyone in politics.

In all our projects on Staten Island, he refused to yield in the face of tremendous pressure. He always insisted on seeing for himself, visiting the facilities, studying up on what Daytop was about. He evaluated the complaints of the protesters with the same thorough attention. And then he made up his mind.

He came quietly to his conclusion that Daytop was an asset to the community. And he stood by us from that moment on, even when it cost him votes. In his own convincing way, he explained to the protesters that they should do as he had done—really look at what Daytop was up to. If they did, he told them, they would agree with him.

That took a lot of bravery for a Staten Island politician. John Marchi is admired and loved for it.

Over the past two decades, few people in public life have faced as much scorn and opprobrium as President Richard Nixon. But let me tell a small part of the other story: On the federal level, no White House has been more caring, more effective, or more intelligent on the subject of drugs than was his. In the years since Nixon left office, he has also become a valued personal friend to Daytop.

While in office, President Nixon pulled together a well-conceived and carefully differentiated drug strategy.

It was under his aegis that the Drug Enforcement Administration was launched, run by the visionary Myles Ambrose. The Nixon administration also played host to a series of very effective White House conferences on drugs. And under Dr. Jerry Jaffee, Nixon turned governmental attention to the whole treatment-prevention side of the drug equation, and he put unprecedented resources there. At the highest levels of government, he expressed a will to attack the problem that has not been duplicated since.

And President Nixon's interest didn't wane when he went into private life.

I will never forget the day in 1988 when he landed in a helicopter on the lawn of our center in Swan Lake, New York.

It was Daytop's twenty-fifth anniversary. He got out of the helicopter, walked across the yard, went inside the house and sat down at the piano. He played "Happy Birthday to Daytop," with seven hundred Daytop kids singing joyously along.

Then, he rose to the platform to speak.

He talked about something that I know must have been difficult for him. It certainly brought his listeners to their feet, applauding and in tears. He recounted some of the difficult moments in his own life, setbacks and embarrassments that he had experienced beneath the glare of tremendous publicity.

"A setback or a defeat in life," he said, "will not be permanent unless you permit it to be. You must rise from your knees and learn from it. You must move on."

Those words just rang across that room, providing extraordinary encouragement to a roomful of drug addicts who were struggling to put their own pasts behind them. This wasn't a show. It was obvious at that moment that Richard Nixon really cared. We owe him a special debt of gratitude.

There have been others. Edward Koch, the three-term mayor of New York, who had opinions on almost every imaginable subject, made time to visit with our kids. So did Senator Alfonse D'Amato, who spoke to the Daytop family about the process of conquering one's self. Another who stands out is Harold Hughes, the former senator from Iowa, a man who became known as the conscience of the U.S. Senate. Hughes was himself a recovering alcoholic, who knew the pangs and the darkness that chemical slavery brings. He served as the voice for those no one cared about and still does, in the creation of the new national organization, SOAR.

Congressman Charles Rangel has distinguished himself over the years for his unusual grasp of the factors fueling America's drug problem and for his unrelenting fight to get Washington to make the right moves. Joining him was Congressman Ben Gilman.

From the health field, we were blessed in New York State with the dynamic and brilliant Dr. David Axelrod, who was commissioner of health until a serious illness forced him to step down. He worked with great compassion on the issue of drug abuse, giving our home state one of the nation's most progressive drug strategies.

We've had help and encouragement from countless figures in the entertainment and sports worlds. They have been generous in sharing their time, their own experiences, and their celebrity status with us. Mary Tyler Moore, who has had so much tragedy in her own life, has been a model of courage for all of us. She loves the Daytop kids, especially the adolescents at our Millbrook center. She even brought her mother and father to visit one of our centers in Italy. All three of them were reduced to tears.

Tony Orlando, the entertainer, has always been there for us, as has been Shirley MacLaine. Down in Texas, the great hero of American football, Roger Staubach, has also been a hero to the Daytop kids. He has been an important role model and is a great booster of bootstrap recovery in life. He lends his leadership to our Texas center.

To these people and a host of others, we owe a tremendous debt.

You might assume that people high in the business world would have little concern about the fight against drugs. After all, they are required to be production oriented and profit oriented. How much could they worry about a bunch of drug-addicted kids?

In more than a few instances, quite a lot.

Some executives at the very top of American corporate life have become wonderful friends of Daytop. They come to visit our centers. They send messages of encouragement and support. They make generous financial donations and convince their friends to do the same.

None of these business leaders is more dynamic than Bill Schreyer, the chairman and CEO of Merrill-Lynch. He heads up Daytop's Executive Council in New York. Tom Cruikshank, who has the top job at Halliburton in Dallas, chairs the Daytop Executive Council in Texas. Both men have become so deeply involved in the work we are doing they are our "Oscar" recipients for their commitment to the young. And John Whitehead is in the front ranks of the caring. The cochairman of Goldman-Sachs for many years and later deputy secretary of state, John was extremely taken by the adolescents at our Millbrook Center. He has stood consistently at our side.

Charles Dyson, a self-made millionaire and a great humanitarian, is another long-standing and consistent friend. He and his late wife, Margaret, turned Daytop into one of their top priorities. So did Bill Wackenfeld, who heads the Hayden Foundation. Bill's concern has translated into many contributions that have enhanced the quality of life at Daytop.

Thankfully, there are others as well, people you'd think would be absolutely consumed by their profit-making enterprises—but, in fact, are never too busy to help with the crises of young people: John Gutfreund of Salomon Brothers; Jerry Junkins of Texas Instruments; Jack Murphy of Dresser Industries; Paul Woolard, the former president of Revlon; Al Shoemaker of First Boston; John McGillicuddy of Manufacturers Hanover; Bill Simon, former U.S. treasury secretary; Bob Abplanalp of Precision Valve Corporation; Frank Smeal of Goldman, Sachs & Company; Nat Ancell of Ethan Allen Home Furnishings; John Mack of Morgan Stanley; Jack Hammack of Hammack Oil; and the late Tom Macioce of Allied Stores are just a few of those who have been splendid to us.

The bottom line for all of them is they dare to care. They stand tall and deliver our message to an American public that is often confused and frustrated. We've all heard so much from the public sector, from government, about the war on drugs. And we see such little result. Thank God for our friends in the private sector.

WHERE TO NOW? **20**

*And this brings out the idea of education, and of Daytop
as an educational institution. It is an oasis, a little good
society which supplies the things that all societies should supply but don't. In the long run, Daytop brings up the whole
question of education and the use which cultures make of
it. Education does not mean just books and words. The
lessons of Daytop are for education in the larger sense of
learning to become a good adult human being.*

—Abraham H. Maslow, Ph.D., *The Farther Reaches
of Human Nature*

Daytop came into being to fill a void. Kids were dying. Families
were despairing. Communities were voicing anger and fear.

Yes, we did intervene. We did create some relief. We did help a
few young people put their lives back together. More than a few,
in fact, and some of them not so young. We brought solace to their
parents and loved ones.

Seventy-five thousand is no small number of lives saved, and the
real number is even greater than that. At the same time we were
helping all those people directly, we put ourselves at the disposal
of hundreds of fledgling treatment programs across the nation and
around the world. If you add up all the broken lives repaired by
those other, Daytop-inspired programs—well, the numbers reach
astronomical heights.

This is obviously a record we are proud of. But it is not a record
for us to lie back and rest upon. If Daytop is to remain a leader in
a national battle against drug abuse, we must never stop asking
ourselves that vital follow-up question: Where do we go from here?

Programs for younger and younger addicts. New ways of reaching
kids before drugs have taken their toll. A better system for inte-

grating education and job training into Daytop treatment. Stronger ties with communities, churches, and schools. Special treatment for pregnant addicts, addicts with young children, and the skyrocketing number of addicts who have come down with AIDS. We came into being to teach people how to live. Now, with the tragedy of AIDS, we are dealing daily with the complex issues of dying, as well.

AIDS represents an extraordinary new burden to an already over-weighted assignment. It was 1984 when I found our beloved Sammy sitting all alone in the dining room of our Far Rockaway Center in self-imposed isolation. He had just been given his "death sentence" by the doctors—AIDS. I took his hand and brought him back to his Daytop family. Everybody was tremendously fearful of this disease in those early days.

The best medical minds were brought to Daytop to lecture. The question was put to the Daytop residents: Abandon or care for the AIDS brothers and sisters? The residents voted overwhelmingly to love their AIDS members twice as much as anyone else, while installing medically recommended precautions. We were all in tears at this decision. Typical Daytop love! And Sammy proceeded to light up our world with his serenity and courage. Sister Mary Francis gave him instruction for First Communion and Confirmation in Spanish, his native language. Bishop O'Keefe confirmed him. And Sammy whispered to me as he fell asleep that night: "I feel so peaceful and close to Jesus." Today, a visitor to St. Peter's Cemetery in rural Liberty, N.Y., would probably wonder about the huge granite gravestone. It carries a simple epitaph: "DAYTOP, WE HAVE LOVED MUCH." Our brothers and sisters with AIDS, by their message of loving sensitivity and courage, have taught us so much about love.

These are just a few of the things we've been working on lately at Daytop. No doubt tomorrow will present us with challenges we cannot even imagine today. We had better remain alive and alert to those.

The evolving social crisis is too severe for us to rest on our laurels, or to be dulled by our honors and kudos. The problems are growing and changing all the time. We must never start to believe—because we have accomplished something and our egos have been nicely massaged—that we are now immune to the prospect of failure. We must not forget that we can still fall short of the mark.

The self-help landscape in America is littered with the failures of well-meaning people who lost sight of that reality. At Daytop, we must never forget the lessons of Chuck Dederich, or those of Bruce Ritter and others. They all succeeded nicely. But they fell victim to their insularity and cockiness, and their successes were sullied by that.

At the same time we keep challenging ourselves to do better, we must keep challenging the world around us. A national campaign against drug abuse is certainly not one that Daytop can wage alone. Thus, that never-ending question—where to now?—is not just for Daytop to answer. It's a question for America, as well.

If we as a nation fail to answer it intelligently, I can promise you we're in for a lot more of the same: more deteriorating communities, more fractured families, more young people addicted to drugs, more violence and, of course, more crime.

Nonetheless, those fraudulent "answers" from the past echo on depressingly. Perhaps we should not be too surprised at this, given our nation's short attention span. But the same old "solutions" are hovering around again, pretending to be bold and new. "Build more jails," the politicians and the editorial writers demand. "Open new hospitals." "Give legalization a try." "Build higher walls along the border." "Bomb Colombia back to the Stone Age."

Sure, the easy-answer crowd has been discredited, time after time after time. But their elixirs are so seductive, you just know they'll be around a while.

There's profit to be made here, after all—of the political and the financial kind. Private hospitals are raking in megabucks, promising those twenty-eight-day wonder cures. Six thousand dollars a week, some of these places now charge. The politicians keep up their pandering, lifting their own careers by exploiting their constituents' pain. All the while, schools are engaged in nonteaching, societies in noncaring, governments in double-talk.

The best response to this avalanche of pabulum, I believe, is to lay out just as clearly as possible those ideas that actually hold promise. That is what we have tried to do at Daytop. That is what I have tried to do in this book.

The answers are really not so complicated, for those who bother to think them through. America can pioneer space travel and fight high-tech wars halfway around the globe. Surely, we have the capacity to formulate an intelligent drug-fighting plan.

But first this nation, which places such value on products and production, must take a deep, hard look at itself. We must put an end to polyester wars on drugs and the other politically motivated cries to the heavens for vengeance. We must all, finally, give some thought to the true meaning of life and to the central values that make life worth living.

Then, we must get on with the business at hand—creating not just a drug-free America but a value-laden America, too. That is a goal worth striving for. It is also, I believe, a goal truly within our reach.

Thankfully, those thirty years of Daytop experience have generated quite a road-map for the trip.

What's called for is a well-balanced, triple-threat attack on drugs—a careful merging of enforcement, treatment, and prevention.

The attack must include all three forces, and they must be released together. Until that happens, our nation's well-hyped war on drugs will remain in shambles. And the human toll will still be there to measure in broken hearts and broken dreams.

Treatment, the main business of Daytop, is the most effective and most immediate way to cut down on the demand for drugs.

In any equation, whether economic or societal, nothing is more paramount than the relationship between supply and demand. The very science of economics is based on supply driven by the engine of demand. One of the truly depressing facts of modern life is how many of our leaders still insist that drug addiction is a glaring exception to this rule.

We have already enumerated the political and self-aggrandizing motivations that have brought us to this impasse, with all its resulting havoc. And yet people still wonder why, in all our wars on drugs, not a single hill has been taken, not a single battle won! It is worth remembering those long-ago gas lines at filling stations in the mid-1970s. The supply cuts in the Persian Gulf were tightening a noose around America's neck. Remember what we did? We addressed demand so as to reduce supply. We installed new hardware in automobile transmissions to increase mileage to the gallon (demand reduction). We launched an energy-awareness campaign tailored to save gas usage (prevention). We changed our lives a little. And it worked. But we continue to ignore the outrageous violation of supply-demand dynamics in the zone of drug abuse.

There are perhaps 5 million drug addicts in America right now and probably another 20 million people who, to one degree or another, are engaged in drug abuse. Many of the casual users will just stop on their own, realizing at some point what a trap drugs can be. But for most serious drug abusers, the first steps toward recovery are extremely difficult to take alone. For them, good treatment programs are truly the only answer.

You really want to cut back on the demand for drugs? Make effective treatment available to everyone who will accept it. This won't merely save the lives of people addicted today. It will save many of tomorrow's users, as well. Those seasoned addicts, don't forget, are the very people who are recruiting others into the world of drug abuse at such an alarming pace.

And what must this treatment entail?

As we have learned over the years at Daytop, it's not enough simply to lock an addict away from the drugs. More fundamental changes must also occur. Otherwise, about fifteen minutes after returning to the street, the average addict will be back on the self-destructive trail of drugs.

Effective treatment must teach basic goals, values and self-discipline. It must be designed for healing the whole person, as well as the entire family—not just the son or daughter who is using drugs. And it must be carefully targeted to the various kinds of drug abusers who need the help.

The population of addicts goes from the minimally to the medianly to the maximally disoriented. Although some of the basic concepts apply across the board, treatment must match the special needs of each and every group.

The first group, the *minimally disoriented,* tend to be younger and just now displaying the early signs of trouble, signaled by declining grades or attendance at school, the appearance of unsavory friends, the onset of intensifying rebellion. Typically, such youngsters don't yet need full-time residential treatment, although many of them will be needing it if their deterioration remains unchecked. This is the clientele that Daytop's Outreach Centers are helping every day. Similarly, services like this must be universally available, and families of these young drug users must be included in the treatment process, as well.

The alternative to such a commitment is unacceptable: generation after generation of young drug users graduating to more severe abuse.

This brings us to the second group, the *medianly disoriented.* Many of them were once in the minimal group, but personal, family, or school denial prevented intervention. They are veteran addicts today, the people that Daytop was founded to serve.

These drug users are genuinely on the skids. They have turned over their lives to drug use. They have mistreated their relatives and friends. Whatever grip they had on education or career has been sacrificed to the heroin or pills or cocaine. If they are lucky, some irresistible pressure—the imminent threat of jail, the horror of homelessness, a particularly persuasive parent or friend—will push them in the direction of treatment. If they are truly lucky, treatment will be available to them.

Most of these addicts need strong medicine, a long-term residential program, like one of Daytop's Upstate centers. Others need shorter terms at Daytop's Brightside Lodge. Almost inevitably, their families are also deeply troubled and they too must be brought into the treatment process. Their parents would benefit from evening therapy sessions. The younger siblings might well be helped by Outreach groups of some sort.

Moving beyond the drug will be tremendously difficult, but with hard work and motivation, treatment can actually work. At those precious moments when addicts can be lured or pressured into treatment, it is nothing less than a human tragedy when treatment is unavailable to them.

Finally, that small percentage of addicts who are *maximally disoriented* can frequently be impossible to reach. They have grown so disaffected, so antisocial, often so psychotic, that drug treatment alone is not nearly enough.

But this doesn't mean that treatment has no role in even these hardest of cases. What is called for in such cases is custodial treatment, a marriage between treatment and incarceration—drug treatment, that is, inside the jailhouse walls.

One of the most creative and effective efforts in this regard is the "Staying out" program at the Arthur Kill Correctional Facility on Staten Island, a therapeutic community inside the prison walls. For ten years now, director Ron Williams has been accomplishing something few prison officials ever do: actually rehabilitating inmates.

Most prisoners, after all, will be back on the streets again one day. Simply warehousing them in prisons in the meantime does neither them nor us any good. It also nearly guarantees problems down the road, while providing "graduate degrees in crime."

We must therefore build into that system of incarceration some incentive to seek treatment. On an experimental basis, Daytop and Daytop-inspired therapy groups have been set up behind prison walls. The results are far from conclusive, but the early signs are encouraging enough.

These days, the criminal-justice system has been given the lion's share of responsibility for fighting the war on drugs. The police and prosecutors and prison wardens get the largest proportion of the dollars and the biggest army of personnel. Their efforts generate by far the greatest media coverage, and the top law-enforcement officials take what are inevitably the grandest bows.

Yet all this activity seems to have done so little good.

All that money, all that fancy equipment, all those expensive guns, all those dramatic seizures: not the slightest dent has ever registered in the supply of drugs on the street.

Is enforcement hopeless? Should the street dealers be allowed to congregate on every corner? Should drugs just be legalized?

The answer to all those questions, I still believe, is the firmest kind of "no."

Although often overemphasized, the issue of supply is still an important part of the drug equation. We cannot afford to ignore it. It's just that the efforts need to be better targeted by far. And they need to be better integrated into a comprehensive drug-fighting plan.

The first step is for the police and prosecutors to get the stars out of their eyes. They have become so addicted to their flashy operations—the high-flying border patrols, the big-weight busts, the film-at-eleven urban drug sweeps—they have lost sight of the truly useful role they could perform. And all of us must help to tear down the giant wall between enforcement, which catches kids, and treatment, which recovers them. Getting "collars" and enhancing police personnel files must give way to a mega-vision of the drug crisis. Cops can no longer afford to be an isolated, adversarial part of society's response to drug abuse. They must stop looking down on treatment as "coddling criminals."

This will take a radical change in thinking and some new operations, as well. The concept of drug treatment must be introduced early into police academies and training centers. The same goes for prosecutor-training programs. The healthy pressure that law enforcement creates on the street is all but wasted today. It must be channeled away from personal or departmental kudos and turned toward recycling rather than warehousing these kids.

The youngster who is exhibiting signs of trouble on the street shouldn't be seen by the neighborhood beat cop only as a potentially "good collar." The cop must see a bigger opportunity than that. By referring the kid to treatment, the cop can save some neighborhood parent a huge bundle of anguish. In both cases, the youngster is gone from the community. Why must it always be behind bars, guaranteeing his quick return to those same streets more dangerous than before? It just doesn't make sense.

In my long experience, the old-fashioned cop mentality only mellows when that officer's own youngster goes on drugs and needs treatment. Why do we have to wait for this? And why is it that police officers, in the military tradition of police work, can opt for a second chance via rehabilitation after falling into the travails of alcoholism but never if the problem is drug addiction? The effect of such shortsighted policies is to drive underground the problem of police officers on drugs. Can't we be smarter than this?

Drug addicts, remember, have a disease that in one important way is unlike all the other ailments that attack the human body. Drug addicts do not *suffer* from their disease. They enjoy it. Their lives may be destroyed by it. Their bodies and their minds may get ruined. But rare is the addict who, in the absence of terrible pressure, will simply decide to give up drugs.

This is the most important role that law enforcement can play. The explanation lies in Freud's pain-pleasure principle. People are drawn to that which is pleasurable. They seek to avoid that which causes pain. Thus, in the war on drugs, the cops and the courts are in a uniquely well-placed position to impose much-needed pain.

But the pressure must be applied thoughtfully. It must be directed where it can really help. And this must occur at the level of the addict and the addict's immediate supply network.

This means local, street-level law enforcement, using the criminal-justice system to pressure addicts to get their lives back on the track. This has obvious, immediate benefits for the people involved. It has long-standing benefits to the society that becomes rid of the addicts' antisocial ways.

By comparison, those DEA agents buzzing Thailand in their airplanes add up to so much wasted time.

The heat that can be applied by local police and judges is often the only thing that brings addicts into treatment at all. "Daytop or jail?" It's not a pretty choice for any addicted criminal defendant. But it's a choice that happens to have brought thousands of addicts into Daytop over the years. It's a tool that should be used more often.

Enforcement, alone, will not cure many addicts. It certainly hasn't taken the drugs off the street. An intelligent program can help create the climate where treatment and, ultimately, prevention can truly succeed.

In the long run, prevention is everybody's goal. It is better for a hundred reasons to convince someone not to use drugs than to arrest or try to cure the person later.

But our national stabs at drug prevention are not cause for much hope.

In the old days, most people wanted to hide from the subject of drug abuse. "That's not something our kids would get involved in," they said. "Don't be planting ideas in their heads." Better to just ignore the growing epidemic and hope it simply goes away.

Eventually, that approach gave way to hysteria. In the film *Reefer*

Madness our children were warned that if they smoked a joint they'd be in hell inside a week. Surely, drugs posed all sorts of genuine dangers. But young people usually know when they are being conned. They discarded the warning as so much hysteria—and then stopped believing even the true things that were said.

In recent years, national drug-prevention efforts have achieved a newfound vogue. Unfortunately, most of them are so naïve, so simpleminded, so cynically devised, they have barely accomplished a thing.

"Just Say No!" How many kids do you think will be swayed by that plea? How silly can you get?

On the prevention side, we need a national drug-prevention program that goes far deeper than the current naïveté. After years of testing various prevention schemes, the country has finally discovered that the efforts must start early. They must reach young people before—not after—they begin experimenting with drugs. Unfortunately, this means elementary school. And the efforts must not let up until early adulthood. The antidrug message must be delivered from all directions—at home, in school, in church, in the media, from every source there is.

But antidrug propaganda, important though it may be, will not do the job alone. The prevention efforts will only connect if they are coupled with real alternatives for a drug-free life. And sadly, many young people have never been allowed to develop such a vision in their minds.

Their families are too dysfunctional. Their education is too disjointed. Their opportunities are too slim. Without the skills for effective living, millions of our young people will continue turning to drugs.

This is a lesson we have learned at Daytop, and that's why today educational and vocational courses are such an integral part of the treatment plan. But even this isn't enough. The other kinds of living skills, the psychological and emotional ones, must also be taught:

how to deal with feelings; how to build relationships; how to create a healthy system of values; how to care for others, how to handle the inevitable setbacks of life.

Teach that to the young people of America. It will arm them with the ability and the inclination to really say no to drugs. It'll do more than a thousand television commercials or a hundred speeches by the First Lady of the United States. It's what real maturity is made of. It's the best insurance there is against future drug abuse.

Treatment to reduce the demand for drugs. Enforcement to put pressure on the supply. Prevention to affect the market future. Those are the elements of the three-pronged campaign. Each has something to contribute to the others. None will work effectively without the other two.

Effective treatment programs, for instance, can be of tremendous help to drug prevention and enforcement by reducing the number of prime infectors on the street, the active addicts who are luring in new converts at a ferocious rate.

In much the same way, enforcement can give a big boost to treatment by pressuring active addicts to commit to change their lives. In the long run, of course, a well-tooled prevention campaign could forestall many of these tragic human descents before they ever occur. But again, you can set up all the life-enriching, family-salvaging prevention programs that you want to. Until they get the reinforcement of safe streets and drug-free playgrounds, until the number of prime infectors is cut, these programs don't have half a chance.

Will all this cost money?

You bet it will, although the ultimate financial cost of an intelligent war on drugs might actually turn out to be cheaper than the current, failed approaches.

Think about how badly we spend the current funds.

Law enforcement's main answer to the drug crisis, for example, is to send addicts to jail. Jail is about four times more expensive than residential Daytop treatment. And it almost never does anybody any good. When Daytop gets done with a resident, that person hasn't been warehoused and forgotten. He or she doesn't return to society with a graduate degree in crime.

Our graduates have grown up. They've learned the values of living. They're infinitely less likely to get into trouble again. And we do all this for a quarter of the price—four for the price of one.

If you add up all the money that is now spent in America fighting drugs, the number falls in the neighborhood of $8 billion a year.

A lot of money, by anyone's count.

Think about some of the other ways we spend money in this country and what we get for them. Just to buy off the bad debt from the failed Savings & Loan Associations, we are spending $800 billion. The defense budget runs to numbers almost that high every year. Space travel. Big weapons. Corporate bailouts. Where do the young people of America fit into the scheme?

We are going to have to put our resources in the areas that have the most claim upon them. Our national defense is obviously important to the future of America. Do the vitality of the family and the lives of the next generation matter less?

We have to start spending the money we have for programs and approaches that are proven to work—not just the ones that generate political dividends. The goal must always be to reverse the horrors of drug abuse, not to advance geopolitical agendas or partisan political gains.

Now, about seventy cents on every dollar of drug-fighting money goes to finance the cops-and-robbers charade: the buy-and-bust operations, the international crop-dust campaigns, the border sentinels, the high-tech surveillance of this or that supposed kingpin.

That is mostly a waste.

We'd be much better off reversing that equation. Put seventy cents of the dollar into treatment and prevention, and thirty in law enforcement, most of it on the local level. We might as well just forget about foreign cocoa-crop rotations, giant fences along the border and high-seas gunfights with drug runners. This merely feeds into the fantasy. There are more drugs on the street corners of America this year than last.

Money isn't all that's needed, of course. Addressing the real issues and the real obstacles will be painful for many of us. It will involve a great investment—not only in money but in sweat, commitment, and time.

But there could be no greater prize at stake, the prize of the American family and especially the prize of its young.

The cancer of drug abuse is eating away at the family's vitality and exploiting all those other problems the family has. If we don't win this important battle, the future of our country will be dismal indeed.

If we don't get started shortly, we may never even get the chance to fight.

INDEX